True Age

CUTTING-EDGE RESEARCH TO HELP TURN BACK THE CLOCK

Dr Morgan Levine

yellow kite

First published in the United States in 2022 by Avery
An imprint of Penguin Random House LLC

First published in Great Britain in 2022 by Yellow Kite
An Imprint of Hodder & Stoughton
An Hachette UK company

1

Book design by Laura K. Corless

A CIP catalogue record for this title is available from the British Library

Trade Paperback ISBN 978 1 529 34489 9
eBook ISBN 978 1 529 34491 2
Audiobook ISBN 978 1 529 34492 9

Printed and bound in Great Britain by Clays Ltd, Elcograf S.p.A.

Hodder & Stoughton policy is to use papers that are natural, renewable and recyclable products and made from wood grown in sustainable forests. The logging and manufacturing processes are expected to conform to the environmental regulations of the country of origin.

Yellow Kite
Hodder & Stoughton Ltd
Carmelite House
50 Victoria Embankment
London EC4Y 0DZ

www.yellowkitebooks.co.uk

True Age

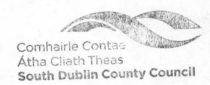

Comhairle Contae
Átha Cliath Theas
South Dublin County Council

To my daughter, Aria, and my husband, Zach. Thank you for filling my days with joy. You help remind me why life is so precious, and I look forward to spending many adventurous and fulfilling decades with both of you.

Age is not measured by years. Nature does not equally dis-
tribute energy. Some people are born old and tired while
others are going strong at seventy.

—Dorothy Thompson, the First Lady of American journalism

CONTENTS

Part I

BIOLOGICAL AGING

1

Contents

Part I

BIOLOGICAL AGING

Part I.

On a sunny April afternoon in Connecticut, I stand in my kitchen trying to make myself salivate. It's my thirty-sixth birthday, and to celebrate, I'm collecting my saliva in a clear tube that I will then place back into its neat little box that will be shipped to a laboratory in Atlanta, Georgia. As my sample begins to rise to meet the black line reading "Fill to Here," I hold it up to the light and examine its contents. I imagine all the cells—a combination of my white blood cells and cheek cells—floating in the frothy liquid. Each one contains a chemical code that can be deciphered to reveal insights into my personal health and aging profile.

As I fasten the cap to the tube and slip it into the bag that was provided alongside it, I think back on all my actions over the past year. Have I been getting enough sleep? Should I have eaten all those sweets over the holidays? What effect will the past year of being in quarantine have— it's April 2021 and COVID-19 has reshaped the world as we knew it. I consider myself to be someone who is very healthy, yet trepidation remains when it comes to peeking under my metaphorical hood. That's because, even though I know I will be blowing out thirty-six candles on my birthday cake this evening, this test will ultimately reveal what my True Age is.

When it reaches the lab in Georgia, scientists isolate my DNA from all the other contents in the sample. DNA is known for containing the genetic code, or set of instructions used to build and maintain each of us. However, it also comprises other critical information buried in a hidden language referred to as the "epigenetic code." Epigenetics doesn't refer to changes in the DNA sequence that each of us inherits from our biological parents (the pattern of A, C, G, and T), but rather chemical tags attached to the DNA and/or the proteins that pack it. These chemical modifications control how our DNA operates or functions. As a scientist working in this field, I refer to epigenetics as the "operating system of the cell." It dictates all the basic functions of a cell, from metabolism to if/when the cell should divide, even down to the identity of a cell. For instance, the neuron cells in your brain have the same DNA sequence as the epidermal cells making up the outer layer of your skin. Yet what sets these types of cells apart is their "epigenome," which instructs a neuron to be a neuron (both physically and functionally) and an epidermal cell to be an epidermal cell. What scientists have also discovered, however, is that the epigenetic code changes as we age, and that by reading these changes, we can determine who among us is aging faster versus slower than expected, and thus reveal our True Age.

A few weeks later I get the email that my results are in. I click on the link, sign in to my personal account, and then scroll down to reveal the answer—thirty-one years old. I am relieved that it's in the direction I hoped—my biological age is five years younger than my chronological age—but to be honest I was kind of hoping it would be better. In addition to my overall biological age score, I am also provided scores for various system-specific measures—things like inflammation, liver functioning, and even brain health.

Given that I was the one who developed these measures, I know that they reflect the age-relative levels of various proteins in my blood that correspond to these distinct categories. For instance, if you were to visit your physician with concerns about your kidney function, the doctor would likely run a series of tests for things like creatinine, alkaline phosphatase, urea nitrogen, bicarbonate. Perhaps you have even had a test like this before. Typically, the numbers would assess various markers and be used to signal whether you might have a disease in the given tissue. But even if you are fine, critical information about your health is hidden within these numbers. By combining them, we can generate your health profile for a given tissue and then use that benchmark to determine whether you appear to be progressing toward disease more quickly or more slowly than is expected for your age. What's more, we don't necessarily need you to take a trip to your doctor or local lab for a blood draw. In fact, we can get a fairly reliable estimate of these profiles from the epigenetic patterns of the cells in your spit.

According to these systems measures, my aging is wonderful when it comes to my metabolic health and brain health. A weak spot appears for me, however, in my immune health and possibly higher levels of inflammation. I am also provided with feedback on what my aging type is. According to the test, around 10 percent of people in the population have an aging profile similar to mine—meaning that they share the same strengths and weaknesses when it comes to the various systems. Generally, people with my profile are more likely to be female, have the lowest obesity rates, yet tend to be at more immediate risk of things like arthritis and even cancer. While it's exciting to learn new things about yourself, what really matters is what you can do about it. Can we "turn back the clock"? While scientists are working to discover ways to slow aging, that doesn't mean we need to sit idly by. There are things each of us can be doing now, and once we "know our numbers," we actually have a way to determine whether the choices we make are helping us.

In this book, I will describe how and why each of us should track our aging, what aging really means, and what we can start doing in our everyday lives to optimize our health. While we don't have all the answers yet, we can take a first step toward achieving a longer, healthier life and reshape how we think about aging.

Beyond Wrinkles:
The Link Between Health and Aging

A s you walk toward the doors of a gymnasium that you vaguely recognize, your hand clasps tightly around your partner's. The early summer heat isn't entirely to blame for your sweaty palms, and you feel your nerves and excitement begin to rise, your heartbeat pounding along with the crescendo sounds of a drumbeat emanating from the open doors. Just outside, a woman sits at a foldout table handing out name tags. As you approach, she smiles, glances at her list, and hands you the white sticker with your name printed neatly on it. "How are you? I am so glad you made it!" she says. "I'm good," you reply reflexively. "It's great to see you too. This should be a fun evening!" As you utter the words, you hope it'll be true—after all, it's your thirtieth high school reunion.

As you enter the gym that is currently masquerading as a ballroom, your eyes slowly adjust to the dim lighting. In front of you are dozens of people talking, laughing, drinking, and a few quickly catching your eye as they assess the newcomers to the party. You can identify many of them, but others cast only a flicker of recognition across your mind—faces you're sure you have seen before but can't quite place. Just to your right, however, is a woman you would know anywhere. She is dancing exuberantly with a small group as they laugh and attempt not to spill the contents of the drinks they are clutching. *It is Maggie, and aside from the hairstyle, she hasn't changed a bit over the past three decades!*

As you start walking over to say hello, you feel someone tap your shoulder. When you turn around, there is a man in front of you, grinning—his arms held up in a *Hey, it's me* gesture. "Wow!" he says. "It is so great to see you! I can't believe it has been so long." Suddenly those nerves you felt earlier in the evening are back. You cannot place the face that is smiling back at you. This man who is probably just shy of fifty years old doesn't resemble any of your former teenaged friends. Thankfully you remember that everyone is wearing a name tag—likely for this exact purpose. You quickly steal a glance down at his. "Wow, Doug! I can't believe it's you . . . You look great!" You hope you are better at lying than name recall, and for a second you worry that the reason you couldn't remember Doug's name was because of some sort of age-related memory loss. *No, that's crazy*, you realize. You're not even fifty. You are healthy as can be, and besides, that won't ever happen to you . . . Or will it?

Suddenly you're struck with the alarming realization that there are surely people in this room who it *will* happen to, and perhaps in the not too distant future. Of your two hundred classmates there tonight, statistics predict that only half of you will survive the next thirty years. Who will make it to a sixtieth reunion? What will you be like if you make it? Will you have more stories to share of loss or narrowly won battles against disease? Will Maggie be dancing as if nothing has changed except perhaps the absence of some much missed friends?

As you scan the room, you realize that you can make a few educated guesses about who will be in attendance. Even though you're only in middle age, it's clear that some trajectories have already started to diverge, accelerating toward the destiny that awaits all of us. Yet for others, time seems to have mysteriously stalled shortly after graduation. Where do you fit? Will you be one of the lucky ones? And is there anything within your power you can do to ensure you see this gymnasium again through the eyes of your eighty-year-old self?

BIOLOGICAL VERSUS CHRONOLOGICAL AGE

Most of us know how many years, and perhaps even how many days, have passed since we were born. But is chronological age really just a number? Deep down, do you know how old—or better yet, how young— you really are? We have all thought about it. As humans, we are innately aware of the changes that seem to coincide with every passing year. We know mortality is imminent and that something about aging slowly draws us toward it.

Time appears to have an inevitable impact on our bodies, our minds, and perhaps even our identities. But while aging is universal, the continuous march of time doesn't intrude on all of us equally. The fleeting years are harsher for some, bringing with them disease, impairment, and loss. For others, the passing of time is only evidenced by the smooth creases at the corners of their eyes, or the indelible remnants of past smiles. The explanation? We all age at different rates and in different ways. While our chronological age may increase at a constant and universal rate, signified by the number of candles on our birthday cakes, the same cannot be said for our biological age, or what I like to call our "True Age." And it is this age that we need to pay better attention to.

Biological age—not chronological age—is what underlies the changes we see in the mirror. The changes we feel as we rise out of bed each morning. The changes that cause most of the diseases and conditions that plague living creatures as they grow old. We have been conditioned to care about our chronological age. To hide it or feel ashamed of it. But the opposite should be true. Our chronological age is a badge of honor. It represents our accomplishments, memories, and the moments spent with loved ones. It captures all the beautiful things that make life worth living. But the best, and perhaps only, way to truly earn more chronological years is by taking up arms against its unfortunate companion—biological age. Luckily, both nature and science have shown us that this is possible to a degree, and that in many ways, you hold the key.

WHY AGING REALLY MATTERS

People often ask me how I became interested in aging. My mother is a professor who studies public policy and works toward improving health outcomes and quality of life for older adults. Her research and outreach help to build safety nets for those whose biological age has rendered them vulnerable to physical, social, and cognitive threats. While this likely influenced my career, I think it was my father and my circumstances growing up that motivated me to dedicate my life to the science of biological aging. As far back as I can remember, I've been fixated on the inevitability of mortality and the realities of growing old. My father was fifty-four when I was born—a retired actor who embraced the role of stay-at-home dad. While he was always active and vibrant, I knew at a young age that he was different from my friends' fathers. When most kids weren't yet contemplating a world without their parents, at seven or eight I was already consumed with the fear that my father might not be around to see me graduate from high school or college, walk me down the aisle at my wedding, or meet his grandchildren. Much to my relief, my father was able to be there for all of these things, including seeing me earn a PhD and be offered my dream job as a professor at Yale University in the School of Medicine. In fact, my father remained in fairly good health for most of his life, up until losing his battle with stomach cancer at the age of eighty-six, two days before I moved from Los Angeles to New Haven to start my position at Yale—a job focused on studying the science of aging.

Most would agree that my father's survival to the age of eighty-six in relatively good health qualifies as a success. But I often find myself lying in bed and contemplating what I wouldn't give to have ten, five, or even one more good year with him. I imagine this is a sentiment shared by most people who lose loved ones to tragic illnesses like cancer, heart disease, stroke, diabetes, or Alzheimer's disease. These surprise losses feel beyond our control. When my dad received his cancer diagnosis, I felt helpless. Yes, we can turn to medical professionals in the hope that some treatment may prolong our loved one's time on Earth, but what we all too often fail to recognize is that the process that put the situation in motion has been unfolding for decades. Perhaps since birth.

This is because all of these diseases are caused by biological aging. It is not chronological time itself that renders each of us more susceptible to disease, but rather the biological changes taking place among the molecules and cells in our body that serve as the foundation from which diseases arise. Simply put, biological aging is the single greatest risk factor for disease and death.

Whenever I teach a class on aging, I start by asking my students what they think the biggest risk factor is for lung cancer. Many assume it's smoking. There is no debating that cigarette exposure has an enormous impact on lung cancer risk. According to the Centers for Disease Control and Prevention (CDC), smokers are fifteen to thirty times more likely to develop lung cancer than nonsmokers. The correct answer, however, is actually "aging." The National Cancer Institute estimates that the risk of developing lung cancer in your twenties is less than 1 in 200,000, yet in your seventies the risk becomes eight hundred times greater. Again, this is not something to do with chronological time. Rather, the lung tissue of a seventy-year-old is inherently different from that of a twenty-year-old. The same goes for nearly every organ, tissue, and cell type in your body. As the years pass, we will diverge from the biology of our former selves. Small changes, driven by damage—or just living—will accumulate in all of us. The rate of that accumulation, however, and thus how far we diverge over time, varies for each of us, and this has a direct impact on our future health and well-being.

While it remains unclear which kinds of aging-related changes pose the greatest threats, in my lab at Yale, we are developing methods that enable us to track many of these changes, with the hope of eventually discovering how to slow or even reverse them. As of now, we can clearly show that individuals who have accumulated more biological age changes than what would be expected based on their chronological age tend to be at greater risk of death and multiple diverse diseases.

Down the road from my lab at Yale sits a modern glass-and-brick building rising high above most of the surrounding structures. This building houses the Smilow Cancer Hospital and the Yale Cancer Center, where, in addition to treating patients, scientists and medical doctors perform cutting-edge research into the causes and consequences of cancer. Through my involvement with the center, I have had the opportunity to develop exciting research collaborations with many of the other members, including two oncologists, Dr. Erin Hofstatter and Dr. Lajos Pusztai. Through this collaboration, our team's goal has been to understand how age-related changes in breast tissue and/or blood impact the risk of cancer. Tracking age-related markers may facilitate prevention or allow us to identify cancer cases much earlier in the disease process.

One of the most common prevention measures in breast cancer treatment is the mastectomy. First performed in 1889 by Dr. William Halsted, it was shown that removal of the tumor and surrounding breast tissue led to a reduction in local recurrence rates. Later, this proved to be the case only for women whose cancer had not yet spread to nearby lymph nodes. Unlike the somewhat barbaric mastectomies of Dr. Halsted's time, today's procedures remove one or both breasts while attempting to spare the skin and underlying muscle.

While this procedure is done to save patients, the tumors and surrounding tissue that is removed can also provide scientific hints into the causes and potential treatments of breast cancer. Through our collaborative efforts, our team of scientists examined the signs of aging in the surrounding breast tissue from women who underwent mastectomies to treat breast cancer, as well as women who underwent elective procedures to remove breast tissue, either as a preventive measure or to achieve reduction. In both cases, we extracted DNA from what is considered the "normal breast tissue," meaning that even in women with cancer, we are not looking at the DNA from the tumor itself. We then used these samples to estimate how biologically aged the breast tissue was—I will expand on how this is done in chapter 2.

What we discovered was that when comparing the biological ages between women with equivalent chronological ages, breast tissue from women with cancer appeared biologically older than the tissue from women without cancer. While one possibility is that having cancer may accelerate the aging process in nearby healthy tissue, we think the more likely scenario is that women who have accelerated aging in their breast tissue may be more prone to developing breast cancer. The same may be true for other cancers—aging-related changes in the tissue can promote tumorigenesis.

We have also shown that this finding is not just specific to cancer. For instance, we looked at aging in brains using the exact same method applied to predict biological age in the breast samples. What we have found is that individuals who have biologically older brains at autopsy (regardless of chronological age) are more likely to be riddled with the hallmarks of Alzheimer's disease. Similarly, when estimating aging in lungs, those with a chronic lung disease called "idiopathic pulmonary fibrosis" were biologically older, and when estimating aging in livers, fatty liver disease was associated with older biological age. Across the board, time and again, biological aging in different organs appears to drive the development of disease. What's more, beyond promoting the progression of diseases that take decades to develop, biological aging may also make us more vulnerable to spontaneous threats—as in the case of viruses.

AGING AND VULNERABILITY

On New Year's Eve, 2019, the Wuhan Municipal Health Commission in China announced that they had observed an abundance of suspicious new cases of pneumonia. This would later be attributed to a novel coronavirus called "COVID-19." Over the ensuing months, COVID-19 grew into a pandemic, spreading across the globe and infecting and killing millions of people worldwide. Unfortunately, what we came to learn was that COVID-19 disproportionately threatened the lives of older individuals. Italy was one of the first countries to show us just how devastating this infection could be for the elderly. With the oldest population in all of Europe and the Americas, Italy saw its death rate skyrocket to over three times the global average, and by the end of April 2020, approximately 14,000 Italians over the age of eighty had lost their lives.

While some viruses are more dangerous for children—as was the case of the 1918 influenza pandemic—many viral and bacterial infections represent a growing threat with age. In the United States, it was reported that 8 out of 10 COVID-19 deaths were in adults sixty-five years or older. While the exact etiology of why severe cases tend to cluster among older individuals is unknown, it is clearly related to changes that occur as a function of our biological aging process. The aging process impairs our body's ability to protect against external threats. We lose our resilience. This is further evidenced by the pattern of increased COVID-19 mortality among individuals with pre-existing diseases of aging—cardiovascular disease, diabetes, chronic lung disease, chronic kidney disease, and liver disease—suggesting that it isn't just chronological age that determined susceptibility to COVID-19 symptom severity and death, but rather biological age. The older your body is, the worse your chances of surviving if infected.

I want to clarify, however, that while many of those who lost their lives to COVID-19 had existing diseases, very few were critically ill prior to infection. This is important because, for many people, the inconveniences associated with protecting those in our population exposed the prejudices that already existed in our society. As people struggled to stay home, watching life as we knew it turn upside down, a troubling sentiment began to take hold. In the *Washington Times*, online opinion editor Cheryl K. Chumley argued in favor of returning the country to normal, citing the argument that "older people die. That's what they do." This justification wasn't reserved for sensationalist media alone, though many people began to question whether protecting the older population from mortality was a worthwhile endeavor. I saw it come up time and again on neighborhood forums or online social media outlets and blogs. Yes, it is true—older individuals are more likely to die in general. Yet what many failed to recognize was that COVID-19 was not simply stealing away the last few days of someone's life; it was resulting in millions of years of life lost. Many of the people who lost their lives to COVID-19 had years—perhaps decades—left to live. Time that could have been spent with loved ones, contributing to society as a whole. Many were perhaps more vulnerable than others because of their age, but they weren't hanging on by a thread, either. Rather, it took a major stressor like COVID-19 to make them lose their firm grip on life.

THE GOAL OF HEALTHSPAN EXTENSION

Given all the ways in which aging can steal your health—or worse, your life—it's no wonder we resist it. But what if growing old doesn't have to be defined by disease diagnoses, prescription medications, hospital visits, and assistive devices? It is possible to grow old in generally good health, without losing the parts of our identities which we hold most sacred. Unlike chronological age, which ticks upward in a predictable repetition, science and evolution have shown us that biological aging is malleable. It can be made to tick faster or slower, in direct response to your genetics—but more important, also your behaviors. Because of the links between this dilation in biological aging and health, it has been estimated that if we could each slow our aging process down by seven years, so that at seventy we had the biological profile of the average sixty-three-year-old, mortality risk from nearly every major disease would be cut in half.

But how do we do this? On a personal level, the first step is getting to know your biological age. Each of us knows our chronological age—the number of years we have been alive—but most of us don't know how we are truly doing on a biological level. Yes, we can make assumptions based on things like our appearance, energy levels, and the feedback we get from our doctors, but is that enough to determine whether our everyday actions are having an impact? Being able to scientifically pinpoint our biological age puts us in the driver's seat of our own health and wellness in exciting new ways. As with our weight on the scale, biological aging is something we can potentially monitor and take proactive steps to change. Knowing and working to improve our biological age will help us live longer, extending our life span. More than that, however, it will help us live in a healthier way, preventing or postponing disease onset and thus extending what is called our "healthspan."

To demonstrate why focusing on aging and healthspan is critical, imagine for a moment that you have a set of stacking blocks, each one signifying a year of life. Moreover, the blocks are different colors, denoting different stages of biological aging:

- Purple and blue blocks represent growth and development (think childhood and adolescence, respectively).

- Green blocks represent what most of us typically experience in early adulthood, characterized by peak physical and cognitive abilities.

- Yellow blocks represent typical experiences of middle age, when perhaps you have slowed down a bit but overall remain healthy.

- Orange blocks represent what we call morbidity, or a time in your life when you have been diagnosed with at least one chronic condition, yet you are still able to maintain independence.

- Red blocks represent a time of more extreme physical and/or cognitive impairment, often due to the acquisition of multiple chronic diseases simultaneously (multi-morbidity). Often, in this stage there is a loss of complete independence and therefore a great reliance on others or the aid of devices to meet the demands of daily living.

In this hypothetical example, let's imagine that the number of purple and blue blocks are set—you can't really get any more adolescent years. In scenario 1, let's imagine that everyone gets the same total number of blocks, say sixty (after subtracting out the purple and blue). This would suggest that everyone had the exact same life span. As I am sure you already figured out, however, there are various configurations of colors that people could have among their sixty blocks. Person A could have 30 green, 28 yellow, and 2 orange, while person B could have 10 green, 20 yellow, 20 orange, and 10 red. Given that orange denotes years spent with disease and red denotes extreme impairment, all of us I'm sure would rather be like person A—having a much larger proportion of our life represented by robust or good health (green and yellow blocks), with only a small fraction of our life spent with disease (2 orange blocks). This is in contrast to person B, who in this scenario quickly transitions to poorer and poorer health and spends a third of their adult life with disease, ten years of which are characterized by extreme debilitation.

Obviously, in addition to differences in the makeup of your block colors, people also differ in their number of blocks. We think of this as your life span. While Elvis Presley may have only received forty-two blocks in adulthood, Paul McCartney has seventy-nine and counting. Typically, the faster you traverse through the colors, the fewer the blocks you will likely receive. Again, however, there are different distributions of colors in everyone's set, and thus, when thinking about life extension, one can imagine different ways to add years of life (i.e., blocks). For instance, one could add red and/or orange blocks, extending the number of years spent with disease(s). Conversely, one could add green or yellow blocks, increasing disease-free years of life.

While I'm sure everyone would reach for the green and yellow blocks if given the choice, unfortunately the medical systems which we have all grown accustomed to and depend on almost exclusively target acquisition of the orange and red blocks—extension of life after disease. Traditionally, doctors are taught to wait for a disease diagnosis to arise in their patients and then optimize treatments that will increase survival, often at the expense of quality of life. Take our health care system's present approach to diabetes as an example. While many people will have their fasting blood sugar (HbA1c) measured during routine physicals, there is often no discussion about disease prevention until a person is diagnosed with borderline diabetes. Usually, if you are below the cutoff, your doctor will say, "Your blood sugar looks good!" But aside from offering reassurance, physicians should also be actively helping their patients keep their levels as far as possible from the magic lines that differentiate nondiabetic from borderline and diabetic. Not everyone below the clinical threshold is equally at risk of developing diabetes in the near future—the further away you stay from the danger zones, the less likely you are to have the aging process push you over the edge into a disease state. What's more, we know that factors like diet and physical activity can improve these numbers, even in "healthy" individuals. Each of us has vast room for improvement when it comes to maximizing our biological health.

The medical system will always need to attend to patients in need of lifesaving treatments. A complementary focus on extending individuals' years of good health (their healthspan), however, will not only improve quality of life, but will also drastically cut health care expenses and the societal burden of disease for future generations. In fact, fewer people may require lifesaving treatments because the population will experience less disease overall.

Sounds great! The question then becomes, how do we achieve this?

The answer is to slow biological aging. Every year you are handed a block, denoting another year of chronological time, yet the color of that block depends on your biological age. In reality there are not just six colors, but rather a spectrum—that is, there isn't one type of green; there is a continuum from blue/green to green/yellow. Next year, when you are handed that new block, wouldn't you like to know not only what color you are getting but also have a say in it?

2

Why to Track Your True Age

I f our ability to live longer, healthier lives depends on our capacity to slow the aging process, then it becomes essential to actually define "biological aging." In both medical practice and in society as a whole, we typically treat chronological age as being synonymous with biological age. This doesn't work when we talk about aging as something that can be targeted or manipulated, however. For all intents and purposes—unless you are the metaphorical person in Einstein's famous thought experiments—chronological time age is the same for everyone everywhere on Earth and is not something we can modulate, whereas biological age varies by individual. Thus, we need to redefine how we think about and track age.

EROSION OF A PERFECT SYSTEM

As a young man, my father was a star athlete. He played football and baseball for the University of Southern California and was in the U.S.

Marine Corps. Yet, as is the case for everyone, as he grew older, he lost much of the physical ability that defined him. By the time my father was losing his battle with cancer, the strength and vibrance that defined him so solidly in my mind was nearly gone. I found myself supporting his weight on my shoulders as I would help him walk from the house to his favorite chair outside. Thinking back, I can't imagine all the innumerable ways his body changed between his years as a college athlete to when he finally passed at age eighty-six. Minute shifts eventually amassed into the major alterations that would reshape the landscape of his being.

One of my daughter's favorite activities is making sand art. While I hold the bottle, she carefully pours the sand in, one color atop the other, producing vibrant waves and streaks. Often, I end up leaving too much room at the top, and as she carries her new works of art around the house, showing them to her father and turning them upside down to admire the intricacy, the colors start to blend. I often wonder whether this is what happens to each of us. When we are young, our bodies are intricately coordinated works of art. Every feature and function is specifically planned to enable us to function—to live. As we age, however, the metaphorical grains of sand slowly shift. Eventually, the plan loses shape. The functioning is lost—and so too is our viability.

Luckily, how quickly or slowly our body diverges from its once youthful form is not predetermined. Things like damage and stress can accelerate it. If my daughter vigorously shakes her bottle, the pattern will be erased faster. If she leaves it on the counter, it will be slower. When it comes to our bodies, every day we are alive, we are encountering things that may shift our configurations: radiation, toxic chemicals, and damaging particulate matter. Tobacco smoke comprises over 7,000 chemicals, 250 of which have been deemed to be harmful and 69 of which are known carcinogens (cancer causing). Inhaling tobacco smoke—whether firsthand, secondhand, or even thirdhand—thus alters nearly every part of our body, from our lungs to our intestines. Even beyond the hazardous factors in our environment, the process of living itself can cause changes to the structure and function of our body. The things we eat, the air we breathe, every chemical reaction in our body—it all has a price.

Yet one of the most amazing things about biology is that, unlike the sand in my daughter's bottle, our bodies have a remarkable ability to regulate, regenerate, and repair themselves. It is an astonishing characteristic of all living things, and in some ways, it's the definition of life. Thus, in addition to damage, the other major factor that contributes to individual differences in the rates of aging is "resilience"—the body's ability to maintain and repair itself. Without these resilience factors, we would never survive to see the light of day, let alone make it to ninety. Living things are in essence self-regulating and self-sustaining systems, what scientists call an "open system," meaning that the system can take in resources or energy from its surroundings and use it to perform specific functions—one of which is preservation.

Because our bodies are open systems, they can put a lot of work into growing and maintaining their very precise structure, and the more efficiently they do this, the more resilient they are to changes. Some individuals are innately more efficient at maintenance than others and, unfortunately, all of us become less efficient as we age. Luckily, there is evidence that our lifestyle choices can boost our body's maintenance and repair mechanisms. For instance, evidence suggests that acute mild stressors actually boost resilience.

Two examples of these acute mild stressors are exercise and caloric restriction (CR). While I'll discuss them both in more detail in Part II of this book, briefly, both of these actions will actually switch on your body's maintenance and repair systems. In essence, the mild stress sends a signal to your body that it needs to toughen up. There is also a limit to the degree of stress that will elicit these beneficial responses, however. In contrast to the responses to mild stresses, very prolonged or extreme stress can actually have the opposite effect, causing widespread damage and accelerating the rate of age-related decline. As with Goldilocks, there seems to be a magic tipping point between beneficial and detrimental stress—it is absolutely possible to exercise too much or eat too little. Thus, the tricky part is figuring out the optimal degree of stress that will increase resilience while minimizing damage. Given that each of us likely has a different optimal level, the best way is to directly measure your body's functioning or degree of aging—to track the effects of various activities on your biological aging process.

PINPOINTING WHERE YOU ARE

Our society has become fascinated with tracking nearly every aspect of our lives. We track our steps, our sleep, our calories, our screen-time minutes, our heart rates; so why don't we track the most important thing when it comes to our health? Perhaps one reason is that people don't have a good concept of what aging is and what it truly represents. Obviously, we all know that being younger biologically is better, but what does it really mean if you're fifty years old according to the calendar, but biologically only forty? To reiterate, biological age represents where someone is on the life span continuum—how much they have diverged over time and how much more they have yet to go before the level of divergence is terminal.

To illustrate this, I often imagine life as a ten-mile-long track that each of us is running. After a given amount of time has lapsed since the start of the race, we can check back to see where everyone is. Let's say that after 30 minutes, 68 percent of the people have completed between 2.5 to 3.5 miles, with the majority being right around the 3-mile mark. Our fastest runner may be at mile 6 and our slowest is at mile 1. While all the runners have been on the track for the same amount of chronological time (30 minutes), they are clearly in different places relative to the start and finish of the race. The next step is to say where we expect the average person to be as time passes. In this case, the average person in our group is running a 10-minute mile—at 10 minutes into the race, we expect them to just be crossing the mile-1 mark. After 20 minutes, 2 miles; 30 minutes, 3 miles; and so on. Using this assumption, we then recalibrate every runner according to this pace. Looking back at our group, which we froze in time after 30 minutes, the people at mile 3 can be said to be 30 (they have run the distance we would expect the average person to run after 30 minutes). Those who are reaching the 2.5-mile mark are 25 (they are where the average person would be after 25 minutes). Those at 3.5 miles are 35. Our fast runner at mile 6 is 60, and our slowest runner at mile 1 is 10.

As I am sure you have figured out, unlike most races, the biological age race is not one you want to win. The slower you are, the longer you get to run the race. Also, unlike an actual race, when it comes to people and their biological ages, it is a little more difficult to tell where they are on the track—we can't just take a snapshot in time and look to see where everyone is. Or can we? Scientists, including myself, are working to develop ways to estimate where a person is on the track at any given period of time. But the way to do this is not clear-cut and there isn't an overall consensus on how to estimate biological age.

Thinking again of my daughter's sand, we can ask how we begin to quantify every minuscule shift that has taken place and altered our resemblance to our former selves. In truth, we can't quantify every age-related change in our bodies, nor do we have to. Instead, we can rely on larger patterns or phenomena. In the case of the sand, this would be akin to measuring things like how far down the bottle the blue sand has traveled, or the change in the width of the pink sand, or the proportion of mixed versus pure colors. When it comes to estimating aging in living organisms, we usually look for patterns in (1) the levels of specific factors produced by our bodies; (2) physical features; or (3) the allotted time needed for the body to complete some pre-specified task.

Interestingly, our brains have already figured out to some extent how to recognize biological aging. When admiring old pictures of our parents, grandparents, or even ourselves, we can easily discern which ones were taken in the teen years, young adulthood, middle age, or old age without having to know the year they were from. That is because our brains are amazingly skilled at recognizing the physical patterns of what defines a young face versus an old face, even if we are looking at the face of someone we have never met before. Some biotech companies are now using artificial intelligence to develop age predictors that, like our brains, can recognize biological aging based on facial images. In general, people who are aging slower overall also tend to look younger. The biological age predictors based on facial images, however, can be discordant when compared to what is happening internally. Things like cosmetic procedures, obesity, and sunscreen habits can make a face look younger or older without also improving internal health.

In my lab, we have been working to develop accurate and reliable ways to estimate someone's biological age using molecular and/or physiological data. This has become possible as a result of huge gains in science and technology when it comes to both measuring biological phenomena and using computers to develop predictions using enormous amounts of data—what we call "big data." As a result, we are able to take a simple blood or saliva sample from an individual and measure tens to hundreds of biological variables that we then combine into a mathematical model to generate an informative estimate of an individual's biological age.

For the majority of people, their estimated biological age is equal to, or at least closely aligned with, their chronological age. Yet for those people who are predicted to be older biologically than chronologically, we have found that they are much more likely to develop age-related diseases like cancer, heart disease, and diabetes in the years to come. We have also found that these individuals tend to have shorter remaining life expectancies. The inverse is also true—individuals with younger biological ages, on average, can expect more healthy years of life ahead of them.

This may make the idea of discovering your own biological age sound daunting, and in fact, when I talk to people about biological age, a response I often get is "I just don't want to know!" The power of biological age, however, is not necessarily to give you a glimpse into your future by telling you how likely you are to survive the next ten to twenty years. Instead, it is meant to give you a glimpse into a possible future—one that you have the power to alter. Your biological age on any given day is not your destiny. It is what we call a "modifiable risk factor." Granted, there are limits (currently) to how young a person of a given chronological age can be biologically. Yet among people of the same age, there is huge variability in biological age, most of which cannot be attributed to genetics. Therefore, in revealing your biological age, we are giving you the insight you may use to take control of your health.

It is the same concept employed in weight management. If you are trying to lose weight, you should know how much you weigh and what your goal is. You need to know your numbers if you are trying to change them. If you don't, how will you know if you are on the right track? This is particularly imperative for young or middle-age adults. Often, people in their twenties, thirties, and forties have no conception of how healthy they really are relative to their peers. It's only after they get older and begin to develop signs of disease that they recognize the fingerprint of aging. By measuring something like biological age early in life, a person can uncover insights that may help them slow their aging process and, we hope, postpone disease onset.

SOUNDING THE ALARM BEFORE IT'S TOO LATE

I was recently asked to estimate the biological age of a thirty-seven-year-old woman named Rebecca. Given that she is young, she has yet to exhibit any signs of disease. She does have a larger-than-normal waist circumference, however, and is classified as obese according to her BMI. When she and her doctor discussed her recent laboratory results, everything was found to be in the normal range according to standard laboratory references. What her doctor failed to notice by looking at her blood tests, though, is that, relative to what would be expected for her age, she is actually quite unhealthy. In fact, at thirty-seven, when I estimated her biological age, it suggested she resembled someone who was actually forty-four years old.

While a seven-year difference may not sound that bad, it is enough to greatly increase her mortality risk, compared to her peers. Among those her age, she ranks in the highest fifth percentile for biological age. Moreover, it is not the mere fact that she is seven years older biologically, when compared to the average person her age, but rather that the divergence in biological and chronological age happened over only a span of thirty-seven years. Let's imagine that at some point in her life, she had an average biological age equal to her chronological age. If the last time that was the case was at birth, we can assume that she was aging 20 percent faster than expected—she aged forty-four years, biologically, over thirty-seven chronological years (the ratio of 44 over 37 is 1.2). If she were to continue on this trajectory, by the time she reaches her sixty-fifth birthday, we would predict that she would have a biological age of seventy-seven. Let's give her the benefit of the doubt and assume she was aging normally up until approximately age twenty-three. In high school she played sports and had the benefit of being young and resilient. After college, though, her lifestyle started to take its toll. Under this scenario, it would suggest that in the past decade and a half, her aging had accelerated to being on average 50 percent faster than expected— over the last fourteen years, she has aged twenty-one years biologically. At this rate, she would be lucky to make it to her sixty-fifth birthday, but if she did, she would have a biological age of ninety-seven and a half years.

In Rebecca's case, we only have one snapshot in time for her biological age, and there is only so much that can tell us. In truth, what we want is continuous feedback of our aging process over time. Just as you wouldn't weigh yourself once in your life, measuring your biological age on a single occasion will only give you a momentary glimpse of where things stand. It is an incomplete picture. Similar to how many of us weigh ourselves every month, or for some, every day, measuring biological age every year will help determine what we call your "rate of aging." With this information you can start to infer where you are headed and also assess the impact of your lifestyle choices.

After learning her biological age, Rebecca began to transition to a plant-based diet and also attempted to boost her exercise. She started out slowly, eliminating meat from her diet, then dairy, and adding in long walks a few days a week. After a year, her biological age was down to forty-two, and we have plans to test it again next year.

The power of biological age comes down to the fact that it is modifiable. Genetic risk cannot be altered, but your biological age can be. Like Rebecca, once you determine your biological age, you can adjust your behaviors and lifestyle in response, and then retest it to provide an indication as to the impact of your choices.

RETHINKING THE CURRENT MEDICAL PARADIGM

At this point you may be thinking, "If I get an annual physical, isn't that enough? Why do I also need to know my biological age?" It is true that health checks are important for early detection of disease (what we call "secondary prevention"). They are not ideally suited for primary prevention, however, which is the prevention of disease incidence altogether.

What's more, we have shown that holistic measures that evaluate the status of your larger system are much more informative measures than the suite of individual lab tests that are typically evaluated. For instance, many of us have likely gone over our results for things like cholesterol and/or blood sugar with our doctors. Traditionally, if you are below (or for some lab tests, above) a certain threshold, then your results are said to be in the "normal" range. The problem with this technique, though, is that many of these cutoffs are chosen somewhat arbitrarily. There is no magic cholesterol threshold we pass through to enter a state of un-health and disease. Even in the normal range, each of us will vary in our immediate risk for disease, in some ways depending on how close we are—high or low—to the cutoff. Obviously, another related factor to consider when evaluating where a person's risk lies is their chronological age. Having high cholesterol is a much more serious indicator that some-thing is wrong if it is detected in a person who is thirty years old versus someone who is seventy. Yet our medical system engages in standardiza-tion of care rather than personalization.

When assessing biological age, we consider the whole spectrum of possible results across multiple tests, and then assess a person's state in reference to either (1) what is expected for someone their age, (2) how different their profile is from someone who develops some disease or who is likely to die in a given period of time, or (3) how different they are from their previous state. As a result, biological age is more about your personal multidimensional profile than any single lab test. A high value on a single measure is usually not enough to greatly elevate a person's biological age. Because biological age is not binary, it is also more rele-vant to tracking. For traditional lab tests, there are usually only two options—normal or elevated. Sometimes you are given a heads-up that you are borderline, but there is still only so much feedback these binary measures can provide, especially when you are still young.

Given the newness of biological age measures, we are still developing a fully comprehensive understanding of what people can do to slow or reverse their rate of aging. Epidemiological (or population-based) stud-ies, comparing people in the general public, have highlighted some key characteristics shared by those who seem to be aging slower—and the findings are not at all surprising. On average, people who rate younger biologically, in comparison to others their age, tend to not smoke, drink minimally, exercise regularly, eat more leafy greens, consume less red meat, get better sleep, and experience less stress.

This makes sense, because we know these things all contribute to a longer and healthier life. Yet, despite these findings at the population level, we still don't know the impact of each on a given individual. It is likely that adopting more of these habits will decelerate aging, but the results may not be the same for everyone. Additionally, the science itself isn't perfect. We still only have a crude understanding of what the ideal diet is or exactly how much and what type of exercise you should be doing.

ASSESSING OUR CHOICES
THROUGH THE LENS OF BIOLOGICAL AGE

Whenever I am at the grocery store waiting to check out, I often glance over the magazine racks decorating the checkout aisle. It is amazing that every week there seems to be a new diet, a new exercise plan, or a new superfood that is touted. Countless books and articles have been written on the optimal ways to exercise, to eat, to sleep—and the ideal approaches to address every disease or health condition under the sun. But how do we ever really know what works for us and what doesn't? Take nutrition science, for example. Every decade the recommendations seem to change. Part of this is because the compositional differences of people's diets is complex. They don't differ in just one way and often it is hard to determine what the key distinctions are that seem to impact health.

The other problem with these studies comes down to how the dietary variables are measured. First of all, most nutritional studies have to rely on self-reports of food intake over short windows of time. It is just too difficult to objectively and accurately track what thousands of people are eating every day for extended durations. Thus, when we study nutrition, we often have to take it for granted that people are honestly reporting what they eat. But we know that, as with weight or age, people have a tendency to bend the truth on occasion. Second, we have to assume that what people were eating during the study period is reflective of their normal dietary habits. I am sure you can imagine if someone told you that you had to keep track of everything you ate for a week and then submit that to a research team, you would probably be on your best behavior! As social animals that are programmed to strive for group acceptance, people often feel pressured to present their best self, even to strangers. Knowing you are being observed will often give you the extra ounce of willpower necessary to say no to a late-night bowl of ice cream or that second beer. Taken together, these are some of the reasons why nutrition recommendations are rife with contradictions. Every study has major limitations that detract from our ability to learn the truth.

Yet another reason nutritional science is messy is due to heterogeneity. What works for one study population, on average, may not necessarily be generalizable to everyone. There is variability. But the only way to assess whether what was reported to reduce disease risk by the most recent scientific publication is to actually test it for yourself. And that requires an empirical outcome measure—like biological age—from which to determine efficacy.

While not a rigorous scientific study in any sense of the word, this was the basic premise for the episode "The Health-Span Plan" from the Netflix docuseries *The Goop Lab*. In the episode, Elise Loehnen, Wendy Lauria, and Gwyneth Paltrow tried three different diets—a pescatarian diet, a vegan diet, and a five-day fasting-mimicking diet created by my colleague Dr. Valter Longo. (In part II of this book, I will discuss Dr. Longo's work in more detail and explain the reasons behind why these diets were selected.) Prior to starting the diets, each woman had a blood draw that was repeated again after they had remained on the diet for a given amount of time. Both blood tests were sent to my lab and used to calculate the women's biological ages before and after this mini personal experiment took place. What we found was that Elise and Gwyneth showed decreased biological age (of about one to two years), while Wendy essentially remained the same. Now, I am in no way advocating that this constituted a valid experiment; instead, it was more of a fun demonstration meant for entertainment purposes. In reality, a few weeks of a different diet—be it pescatarian, vegan, or a one-off fast—will not have much appreciable long-term impact on health. I would bet that a few weeks back in their normal routines would obliterate any effect we saw in response to the new diet. That being said, it does provide a simple illustration for the application of biological age in tracking more sustained health behaviors.

BIOLOGICAL AGE BIOHACKING

Continually tracking biological age over time on an annual or semiannual basis enables the estimation of a person's rate of aging, which, as I explained before, is far more informative than knowing your biological age at a single point (or even two points) in time. Being armed with the knowledge of our own rate of aging can help each of us develop personal regimens, diets, and routines specifically tailored to keeping us as biologically young and healthy as long as possible—both inside and out.

In many ways, biological age tracking is akin to data-driven biohacking. Generally, biohacking is described in two ways—the first is DIY biology, or essentially amateur labs (e.g., people experimenting on themselves with things like gene editing or drugs). That is not what I am promoting here. The second type of biohacking is based on personalizing health; it is about understanding your own biology to a point where you can optimize it via interventions that are tailored specifically to you and your body. The key to this idea of biohacking is the emphasis on personalization, as well as the individual's accountability in actively promoting their own health. Each of us has a specific health profile and unique biological age measures that we can often alter with simple lifestyle choices and changes. In summary, your health is specific to your own biology and cannot be treated as a "one size fits all" solution.

Measuring biological age will provide individuals with a peek behind the curtain to reveal their unique aging processes and, in so doing, pave the way for each of us to live longer and, most important, healthier lives. Success, however, hinges on a clear definition of exactly what it is we are trying to optimize. If it is to slow aging and improve health—two seemingly abstract states—then how do you determine whether your diet or exercise plan is the best fit for you personally?

After the *Goop* show aired, I received hundreds of requests from people asking if I could measure their biological ages. Many people sent descriptions of what they had been doing in an attempt to slow aging and were desperate to figure out if it was working. Others described their grandmothers who were healthy and thriving at age one hundred and wondered whether they too were blessed with longevity genes. Others confessed their worries regarding their family histories of heart disease, diabetes, or other afflictions, and their goal was to avoid the same fate.

In the past, these individuals would have been out of luck. There traditionally hasn't been any validated way for the average person to assess their biological aging profile. But that's changing. Over the past year or two, a number of consumer-based products have been launched that enable anyone to track their underlying aging and health. These include at-home tests, detailed assessments, or even online surveys that promise to help you get at your true age. Most of the tests will predict a biological age that you can then contrast with your chronological age to determine if you are aging more quickly or more slowly than expected. Some of the tests I have helped develop can provide even more information regarding which systems may be contributing to a higher or lower biological age (more on that later).

While these tests are not all equally valid or reliable, many of them are based on extremely sound science. Yet, before we can assess which measures are the most valid estimates of a person's true age, we first need to define what it is we are actually trying to measure. What is "biological age"?

3

What Is Biological Aging?

The definition of "aging" in the *Merriam-Webster* dictionary is "present participle of age," in which age can be defined as "the length of an existence extending from the beginning to any given time." To me (and perhaps to you as well), this is not a satisfying definition. Aging is so much more than the passage of time, as I hope I have already convinced you. But it is also not clear what would be a more appropriate definition.

If you were to ask a dozen people what aging is, you might end up with as many different answers. In fact, for fun, I surveyed some friends and family to ask how they defined biological aging. Here are just a few of their responses:

> "Gray hairs, wrinkles, being tired . . . and pulling a muscle by turning around when your kid asks you to look at something."

> "It's a syndrome driven by the lack of self-repair mechanisms to effectively correct 100 percent of damage accumulation, error, and dysfunction."

"A synchronized, protracted shutdown that depends on the organism for timing."

"Relegating our meat suits to the vicious deterioration in durability, mobility, and activity that comes with problematic biology."

"The gradual (usually) growth then decline in cells, organs, systems, and function over time."

"A decrease in physical abilities, but an increase in spiritual and emotional and awareness attributes."

"Aging is when the 'finish line' gets real."

"Time with a heartbeat."

IS AGING DESTINY OR CHANCE?

In a small hotel meeting room in New Mexico, a group of scientists—me among them—gathered to discuss mechanisms that regulate aging. Talks about new findings showed how declines in stem cells caused aging. Others pointed to the role of telomere shortening. Although each presenter proposed a different explanation for why we age, one thing every speaker had in common was that they were operating from the viewpoint that damage accumulates over time and that this produces the diseases and functional declines we associate with aging. That is, until the last speaker ascended the podium. This scientist asserted that aging is programmed in our genes. That we all have an internal clock that is actually forcing our body to age, slowly counting down our remaining days. He suggested that this clock was selected by evolution. That aging and mortality are beneficial for the population as a whole, and in short, older individuals die to ensure successful continuation of new generations and to guarantee survival of the group. If true, he suggested that by identifying the central regulator or switch that controlled this progression, one could simply "flip" it off and ultimately halt, or possibly reverse, the process of aging. After all, development is a highly programmed process that can be experimentally manipulated, so why not aging?

Needless to say, this assertion prompted a clamor of rebuttals from the other scientists in the room. They argued that aging is unlike development and that evolution does not optimize fitness of the group over that of the individual. Conversely, we know that our bodies incur a tiny amount of damage every day, and after decades, this accumulates to a level that causes cellular and tissue decline. Essentially, they posited that aging is the price we ultimately pay for living. While I have seen many scientific debates, none sparked as much fervor as those arguing whether aging is a pre-specified program or an unfortunate cost.

My definition of aging somewhat blurs these two opposing sides. I define aging as a "loss of specificity." I believe that there is a specific state—or a small number of states—a body can have that is optimal for health (think back on the example of the sand art). Achieving and maintaining this state, however, requires a lot of work on the part of the body. It's not an easy task. Through evolution, our bodies have "learned" how to efficiently and reliably reach this state—development is extremely precise and has programmed steps to ensure that it is successful for the majority of us. That's the whole reason we are here. Luckily, we have one of the developmental programs that works well. Species with far inferior developmental programs are not represented among living things. They cease to exist because they are incompatible with survival.

At the same time, I do think species' life spans are to some extent programmed, but only insofar as they are set up to counteract aging. This is distinctly different from the way we think of programming in development. In aging, it is the strategy to oppose that is programmed. Aging itself is the default. It is not something that has to be spurred on. Imagine a hill, the top of which symbolizes that ideal state that epitomizes health. Development represents a ball ascending the hill, while aging, descending. It takes energy to roll the ball up the hill. A program must be in place to make sure energy is taken in and efficiently used to reach the crest. Similarly, it also takes energy if you want to slow the descent down the other side of the hill. But nothing is needed to ensure the ball can roll down the hill once it starts. It will do it on its own without additional force behind it.

While evolution has perfected a strategy for getting the ball to the top (development), there is no evolutionary pressure to optimize maintenance of this state for longer than what we currently observe. Completely preventing aging is not evolutionarily advantageous—the benefit does not justify the energy cost. Remember what you learned in your high school biology class about genetics. Whether a trait is selected for generally depends on its effect on fitness. Also remember that fitness in this case is not defined as the strength of the individual (that is, how fast you can run from a lion, as it is commonly misconstrued), but rather the number of reproductive offspring one produces (although if you can't run from the lion . . .). Thus, there is no evolutionary benefit to putting in a lot of work to maintain a body past when it is either (1) still able to reproduce, or (2) its continued survival is beneficial to the survival and reproductive fitness of its offspring. Once an individual has exhausted their fitness capacity, there is no cost to allowing nature to take its course. The ball is permitted to roll down freely. While evolution may see us as disposable once we pass our reproductive prime, most of us don't share this sentiment. Luckily, there is substantial evidence to suggest that the rate of biological aging is malleable—the ball's descent can in fact be slowed.

Thinking back to our hill metaphor, we find there are two things that can be programmed which will alter the length of time it takes to descend the hill—i.e., the rate of aging. First is the distance to the bottom. The farther you have to travel, the longer it tends to take. While the hill is an analogy, I like to think of this distance as representing something about the robustness, resilience, or complexity of the individual in their optimal state. It takes longer to unravel an intricately designed and reliable system than it does a simple one. The other thing that will have a clear impact on the time it takes for the ball to descend to the bottom of the hill is the energy/friction/force used to oppose its descent. As mentioned in chapter 2, our bodies can utilize energy to counter age-related declines.

THE NATURAL DIVERSITY OF AGING RATES

We know that different species have different programmed mechanisms for repairing or preventing damage and decline. Probably the greatest demonstration of this is the profound diversity in life span across the animal, plant, fungi, protists, and bacteria kingdoms. It's amazing that living things are more or less made of the same "stuff," despite there being enormous variation in how well that stuff holds up over time. As one of my neighbors said, "I'm still mystified by different aging rates. For example, why do dogs get cataracts at eight years old? Or arthritis by twelve? Isn't the raw tissue, bone, and so on basically the same stuff? Muscle is muscle. Eyes are eyes. It's to do with the overall design of the organism rather than tissues wearing out. Almost as if tissues, et cetera, wear out in anticipation."

There is no denying how amazing it is that nature uses the same essential building blocks to make up so many diverse species with drastically different life spans. On average, 85 percent of protein-coding genes in the human genome are identical to that of a mouse, but we live forty times as long. And neither the mouse nor the human is even close to the extremes.

Slithering across a plate of gelatinous material derived from red seaweed, the roundworm represents one of the most popular invertebrate animals in biology labs. This worm, named *Caenorhabditis elegans* (*C. elegans*), contains approximately a thousand cells in total and has nearly as many genes as we do. Yet, unlike us, the worm can produce nearly three hundred offspring over its very rapid life span of only two to three weeks.

On the other side of the spectrum, the Greenland shark, weighing in at more than a ton and spanning up to fifteen feet in length, is the longest-lived vertebrate on the planet. This slow-moving fish cruises the cold and dark North Atlantic and Arctic waters. While precise estimates of their life span had long eluded scientists, in 2016 a paper was published that examined lens crystallins in the eyes of Greenland sharks. By measuring how much carbon-14 was contained in them, the scientists were able to carbon-date the sharks, suggesting that they lived nearly three hundred years on average, and did not meet reproductive maturity until age a hundred and fifty.

Even more perplexing yet is the diversity in life span within species. Since we moved from the dry Southern California climate to a large lot in rural New England, one of my beloved summer and spring activities with my daughter has become gardening. While tending to the perennials, we admire all the creatures we encounter, from butterflies to earthworms, and even the honeybees. The honeybees are my favorite, not just because of their important standing as the world's most essential food pollinators, but also because they represent a perplexing model of aging.

Within the honeybee colony reside three castes—the drones, the workers, and the queen. The drones are the male bees, whose sole responsibility is to mate with the queen. The average life span of a drone bee is eight weeks. They often die within hours after successfully fulfilling their duties, or else are killed by the workers, given their drain on resources. By contrast, the females—the worker bees—enjoy longer life spans. In the winter, the worker bees can live an average of five months or more. And this pales in comparison to the two- to five-year life expectancy of the queen bee.

The difference in longevity between the male and female bees may be driven by genetics. Unlike humans, the drones have half as many chromosomes as their female counterparts. But genetics does not explain the difference between the workers and the queen, as they have nearly identical genomes. Thus we can rule out the possibility that the queen was endowed with a longevity gene that somehow slows the rate of her demise. Rather, the difference comes down to how environmental signals become coded in their biology. As larvae, the future queen and her underling sisters partake in dramatically different cuisines. The larva queen feasts on "royal jelly" secreted from the glands of her nurse bees. Meanwhile, the prospective workers enjoy "beebread," composed of fermented pollen and honey. While there is a debate over whether the royal jelly imbues the future queen with her royal traits, or if the beebread robs the workers of their queenly potential, one thing is for sure: when it comes to female honeybees, diet has the potential to increase longevity four- to tenfold.

READING THE TEA LEAVES OF EVOLUTION

Given the vast differences in life span both between diverse species and among genetically identical siblings, scientists have speculated that by determining the causes for such diversity, we could in essence hack the system to reengineer what evolution has already demonstrated is possible. Unfortunately, this is easier said than done. It is unlikely that there is a single factor that governs life span differences. Instead, the more plausible scenario is that there are thousands of differences between short-lived and long-lived species that have been acquired over eons.

But what about the case of the honeybee queen? She has the same genome as her worker sisters—no gene editing needed—but she lives more than five times as long. There is no saying whether a similar system could be manipulated in us to extend our longevity. Is it possible to discover the human equivalent of "royal jelly"? I don't know. The important takeaway, however, is that this goes to show that the rate of aging is highly malleable and may not require gene editing (or changing what it means to be human). Like the honeybee, our bodies are programmed to alter their functioning based on inputs from the world around us. This includes signals from our lifestyle, behaviors, physical environment, and even psychological states. By figuring out how the body responds to the outside world and to itself, we may be able to increase healthspan and life span, but to what end?

Nobody knows whether there is a limit to human life span. On one hand, some argue that there are no laws suggesting open systems have to age, which is true. On the other hand, however, the manner in which the human body is structured and programmed may limit its capacity for longevity far beyond what has been observed. Regardless, the goal of aging research should extend beyond the quest for immortality. The ability to improve upon our innate maintenance and repair mechanisms would be a huge win. As mentioned in chapter 1, most people develop disease in their sixties and may survive another twenty years. But imagine living to one hundred or beyond in good health and then slowly declining over the remaining five to ten years. That is ideal, and that's what our goal should be.

While scientists around the world are diligently working in labs trying to decipher what signals control the rate of aging, figuring out how to accomplish this feat is incredibly difficult. Even if we discover a way to slow aging, it will likely require constant work to maintain, especially for complex organisms like people. There won't be a magic pill you take once and then poof—you're a super ager. Yet despite the uphill battle we face, trying to intervene in biological aging is a valuable endeavor.

Personally, I consider the significance of healthspan extension to be so great that I have devoted my entire career to the cause. Given the complexity of biology and the aging process, I imagine it is something that I will spend my life working to understand. While I am perhaps less optimistic than some of my colleagues that the keys to major healthspan and life span extension are just around the corner, it is also amazing to look back at all the work that has been done in this field to understand what happens to our bodies as we age.

WHAT HAPPENS WITH AGING— FROM THE BOTTOM UP

When we talk about the myriad changes that occur with aging, it is important to keep in mind that biological systems (like humans) are composed of different levels of organization. The smallest level is the atomic level, followed by the molecular, cellular, tissue, organ, organ system, and organismal (whole body) level, in that order. Technically, the levels continue—population→community→ecosystem→biosphere—but for the sake of this book, I'll mainly be discussing the molecular through the organismal level.

Most scientists agree that aging likely begins at the level of molecules and then propagates upward, eventually becoming evident to the individual once it reaches the tissue/organ and then organismal level. So, let's start at the bottom and metaphorically shrink down to 1/20,000th the diameter of a strand of hair. At this size, we would be slightly taller than the average protein in our body.

Proteins are often referred to as the building blocks or the body's workhorse. They make up a large portion of our physical structure and perform a wide range of essential jobs needed to maintain life. For instance, structural proteins, like collagen and actin, make up much of the foundation of many of our tissues, including what's called the "extracellular matrix." Imagine the layout of a city. The extracellular matrix would be the roads, bridges, and property lines, as well as power, water, telephone, and sewage lines. It dictates the layout of the city (the tissue/organ) and the density of homes and buildings (cells), and facilitates transfer of goods, energy, communication, and waste.

In this molecular city, we will also find a plethora of other proteins that help ensure everything operates correctly and efficiently. There are the delivery trucks (transport proteins) that supply essential goods like oxygen, cholesterol, or sodium to cells all around the city. There are police officers, who are akin to defense proteins, like antibodies. Their job is to survey the area in order to protect us from invading pathogens. The phone lines and cell towers (signaling proteins) serve as the basis of cell-to-cell communication. The market (regulatory proteins) dictates supply and demand of products and drives the rate of production. And finally, the workers (enzymes) make everything run and are active participants and catalysts for all that happens in the city. Without them, nothing would transpire—no production, communication, shipment/delivery, and so on.

When it comes to the various proteins in our body, their ability to perform any one of these given tasks is dictated by their structure/shape. A central idiom in biology is "structure determines function." Thus, like beautiful origami art, each protein made in our body is folded into a specific intricate 3D structure that will enable it to perform its intended purpose. Unfortunately, one thing that happens as we age is that structures become compromised. Proteins with errors in their sequence are folded incorrectly, inhibiting their ability to perform their specified tasks. Yet even those that are compiled with the correct sequence can undergo chemical modifications after they are created. These modifications, called "posttranslational modifications," can alter the protein structure and function. With aging, the excess presence of things like reactive oxygen species, sugars, and/or fatty acids can attach to and modify proteins. In some cases, these misfolded or modified proteins will link or clump together, forming larger structures that can damage nearby tissues or cells, and are difficult to break down and clear.

Thankfully, our bodies have evolved mechanisms to detect and replace problematic proteins. Every cell in your body has a recycling center that targets and degrades damaged proteins and then recycles their parts. Unfortunately, like the proteins that lose functional capacity with age, so too does the system that was set up to deal with them. This efficiency of the recycling program and the initial propensity for proteins to become damaged in the first place does seem to be responsive to lifestyle, to some extent. Damaging agents—such as cigarettes, air pollution, or foods high in sugar or trans fats—can exacerbate the misfolding of proteins, while exercise or other mild stressors can ramp up the body's recycling conveyor.

EPIGENETIC AGING

Beyond proteins, another age-related molecular alteration that I have spent considerable time studying is the change in something called "epigenetics." At the beginning of this book, I described a test I was taking that used epigenetic information to estimate my biological age. To recap, epigenetics does not refer to changes in your DNA sequence, but rather the addition or subtraction of various chemical marks to the DNA structure or the proteins that DNA is wrapped around. These chemical tags directly influence the shape of packaged DNA, dictating which sections can be accessed and which cannot.

In many ways, epigenetics is the recipe book for your cells. The genes and the resulting proteins can be thought of as raw ingredients. Each of your cells has the same ingredients—the same DNA sequence. But the epigenetic patterns are what determine which ingredients are used. Certain cell types will use certain ingredients and alter the levels of other ingredients. This is all dictated by the epigenetic pattern in that cell and is carefully planned out to optimize functioning of the system as a whole. Just like with proteins, each cell has a specific role and thus it is critical that they have the right epigenetic recipe to achieve it. Unfortunately. the epigenetic patterns in cells are impacted by aging. Things are incorrectly written or erased, and all of a sudden, we have the wrong recipe. Our cells end up generating too much of one protein, not enough of another, or have an entirely different recipe altogether—causing them to lose their original identity.

While the direct cause of these epigenetic changes is not known, one hypothesis is that they reflect random errors. As cells make new versions of themselves, they copy both their genome (DNA sequence) and their epigenome, so that the new cell is a perfect copy of the original. It is thought that perhaps not all the epigenetic marks are copied over correctly, and new evidence is surfacing to support this idea. It has been shown that both in cancer and in aging, the areas of the genome that tend to show altered epigenetic patterns are those in what are called "late" or "early replicating" regions.

When a cell is ready to divide and make a new daughter cell, it will unwind its DNA so that it can be copied. This process is called "DNA replication." Replication doesn't happen all at once across the entire genome, however. Instead, cells have a replication timing program that dictates which regions are copied, and in what order. Typically, the regions being used most by the cell are copied first and then ones that are completely turned off are copied last. Research is showing that these two opposite regions are the ones that become the most dysregulated with both aging and in cancer—which is a problem. If all of a sudden the regions that should be off get turned on instead, and vice versa, the recipe will be a disaster and the cell won't operate as expected.

In fact, my lab has been able to show that by simply letting cells divide in a dish, we can observe the same epigenetic changes that we see in people's (or animals') bodies with aging. As cells divide, their epigenome becomes less and less like the original "blueprint." Eventually, these changes will influence what proteins are synthesized and, in some cases, could even affect the production of important factors like tumor suppressors, whose job it is to help guard against potential cancer-causing events. Similarly, another potential consequence of age-related epigenetic changes is a loss in repression of ancient viral genes, called "transposable elements," that have become permanent fixtures in the genomes of humans (and other organisms). Discovered by Dr. Barbara McClintock in the 1950s while studying genetics in corn, the spontaneous mobilization of transposable elements has become a major focus in aging science. One major role of epigenetics is to silence these genes. Nonetheless, as errors in the epigenome accumulate, retrotransposons can become activated and wreak havoc on the cell.

While many of the epigenetic changes we observe with aging may be due to random errors, or bad luck, another possibility is that some of these changes represent the cell's response to a failing system. Due to the changing environment around them—the breakdown of the structural proteins that house cells, signals from their distressed neighbors, and the accumulation of toxic by-products—cells may choose to change their behavior as part of a programmed stress response. Evidence of this has come from the incredibly compelling data showing that the epigenome can be reprogrammed (or reset) to mirror a young epigenome simply by introducing various factors into the environment. It is possible that cells that have acquired random errors simply "remember" their initial blueprint and can restore it when signaled to. Another possibility, however, is that the changes we observe in the epigenetic pattern are simply a response to something in the aged environment, and that they can be turned off or reversed under the right conditions.

While we are still trying to understand why these changes occur, an important observation we have made is that individuals whose cells appear to have undergone more epigenetic changes are at more immediate risk of various diseases. Similarly, many of these same epigenetic patterns are observed in cancer—just to a greater degree. While cancer biology is built on the concept that a cause of cancer is the accumulation of random mutations that occur when the DNA is replicated, some researchers are also starting to look for potential epigenetic causes. These may also explain why the risk of developing cancer in a given year rises exponentially with age. Given that the epigenome is prone to imperfect copying that accumulates with age, these changes may explain why old cells are more likely to become cancerous. It also presents another possible explanation as to why tissues that naturally divide at faster rates are more prone to developing cancerous tumors. Without intervention, cells may have a limit as to how many times they can divide and still remain viable and productive members of a tissue.

LIFE SPAN AND AGING OF A CELL

In 1881, a German biologist by the name of August Weismann suggested that "death takes place because a worn-out tissue cannot forever renew itself, and because a capacity for increase by means of cell division is not everlasting but finite." Eighty years later, Leonard Hayflick and Paul Moorhead would publish a paper effectively validating Weismann's hypothesis. While they did not show it to be the root cause of aging, Hayflick and Moorhead showed that cells in a dish have a limit on how many times they could divide. This would come to be known as the "Hayflick limit," and remains ingrained in our scientific thinking even today, sixty years after the initial discovery. Not long after Hayflick and Moorhead's discovery, it was shown that the likely explanation for this limit was a phenomenon in which a DNA sequence becomes shorter with every cell division. Specifically, the trailing ends of the chromosomes, called "telomeres," cannot be copied fully due to how the replication machinery is configured. Every time a cell divides, a little bit is left off the end. Telomeres are often alluded to as being like the protective plastic caps on the ends of shoelaces, and while I don't agree, some scientists have speculated that their progressive shortening may be the root cause of aging.

Yet despite the Hayflick limit, our bodies do have mechanisms to guard against telomere attrition. In a lab at the University of California, Berkeley, in 1984, a young professor named Dr. Elizabeth Blackburn and her graduate student, Dr. Carol Greider (now a professor of molecular biology and genetics at Johns Hopkins University), discovered the protein telomerase. Telomerase adds base pairs (the ACGTs) back to the end of one of the strands of DNA so that the original strand can be copied in its entirety. Thus, telomerase is essential for counteracting the threat of telomere shortening and preventing the cell from realizing its Hayflick limit. Initially, this was viewed as a potential key to solving aging. If telomere shortening explains why cells lose the ability to replicate and thus regenerate aging tissue, then all we have to do is maintain the telomere length so that the cells can go on dividing as normal. But like everything in life, if it sounds too good to be true, it probably is! You see, telomerase activity is one of the major hallmarks of cancer. It is what enables cancer cells to continue to divide indefinitely, making them essentially immortal. Therefore, it is believed that artificially increasing telomerase activity in cells that have already acquired many of the epigenetic modifications and mutations that accumulate with aging would inadvertently be causing cancer. You would be bestowing "bad cells" with the power to continuously divide and make more bad cells.

If you were ever a comic book fan, you will recall that many of the heroes and villains of the DC and Marvel worlds didn't start off with supernatural traits. Instead, they acquired their characteristics through a transformative event. The same could be said of cells. As they experience some of the molecular changes described previously, they may acquire new traits. Some of these traits are beneficial, which is why we have evolution, but others are deleterious. These transformed cells can become the villains in our bodies. Cancer cells are an example of this. They develop from normal cells that by some means acquired additional traits that over generations eventually enabled them to realize immortality,

51

turn off input from neighbors, evade fail-safes that instruct damaged cells to undergo cell death, sequester large blood supplies and energy sources, and eventually migrate and colonize other tissues.

Luckily, our bodies have evolved a fail-safe for preventing altered cells from becoming cancers. If a cell has acquired DNA damage or other changes that may make it prone to transforming into a cancer, a program can be enacted that essentially halts that cell's progression. Instead of morphing into a cancer cell, it becomes what is called a "senescent cell." Cellular senescence is a stress-induced state, usually triggered by things like telomere shortening, DNA damage, or stress signals from neighboring cells. Unlike cancer cells, a senescent cell cannot divide—because they are supposedly damaged, their ability to divide and make more copies of themselves is turned off. Like cancer cells, however, senescent cells are hard to kill. They have mechanisms that prevent them from undergoing cell death and instead just stick around in a state of limbo. For this reason, some people describe them as "zombie cells." They aren't dead, but they also aren't "all there." While this alternative state is a great way to prevent damaged cells from becoming cancerous, it brings with it its own problems. In general, senescent cells aren't just benign beings that insist on sticking around. Many of them are actually toxic.

In addition to losing the ability to divide while evading cell death, most senescent cells also begin eliciting a very specific behavior. Unlike normal functioning cells, senescent cells chronically activate pro-inflammatory genes, leading to prolonged and widespread inflammation. This inflammation can contribute to ever-increasing molecular damage, which in turn can make neighboring cells more prone to becoming senescent or even cancerous. As senescent cells accumulate in tissues, this creates a self-perpetuating cycle of dysregulation. The conversion of normal cells to senescent cells also means that there are fewer cells that are dividing and repopulating tissues.

When we are younger, cellular death and/or transition to senescence is not such a big deal. Our bodies are equipped with sufficient backup stores for replacing lost cells. Enter stem cells. Stem cells supply the resources for replacing lost raw material. There are a number of different kinds of stem cells. Adult stem cells are present in small numbers in a range of organs, including bone marrow, muscle, certain parts of the brain, liver, skin, and so on. They reside in what's called the "stem cell niche" and generally have two main functions. They can divide to create more stem cells (a process called "self-renewal"), or they can transform into specific cell types to replace lost cells in tissues (a process called "differentiation"). For example, as the protective surface of our body, our skin copes with constant wear and tear. Epidermal stem cells thus serve as potential replacements that can differentiate, or convert into mature cells, to replenish the lost cells that form the top layer of our skin (the epidermis). As you can imagine, though, the supply of adult stem cells is not endless.

In the aging process, we observe a decline in the number of available stem cells, which in turn contributes to an impaired ability to replace the lost or damaged cells in our tissues. Stem cells themselves can also acquire some of the damaging molecular changes described previously, causing them to become dysfunctional. Often, these changes will impair the stem cells' ability to undergo self-renewal (make more stem cells) or differentiate (convert into a specific type of cell). In some cases, age-related mutations of epigenetic changes can increase a stem cell's self-renewal.

When this happens, these "damaged" cells will be faster at making copies of themselves and thus causing them to in some ways take over the stem cell pool. This evolution at the cellular level produces a population that is biased toward cells with the specific mutation, a process that has been studied to a significant extent in the context of aging in white blood cells. For instance, researchers have found that stem cells with very specific mutations become more prevalent with age among immune cells. In fact, by age seventy, approximately 10 to 20 percent of people will have detectable white blood cell mutation in a small number of specific genes.

This suggests that these cells may have arisen from overrepresented stem cell "clones." While we don't know the precise mechanism, scientists have linked the presence of these clones to an increased risk of developing a number of major diseases in the near future, including, interestingly, cardiovascular disease. What this suggests is that evolution and selection at the cellular level may actually drive some of the age-related changes we see at the organismal level.

NATURAL SELECTION IN THE CELLULAR WORLD

Recently, when discussing these concepts with a good friend and colleague of mine, Dr. Kenny Beckman from the University of Minnesota, he brought up a paper by the brilliant British physician and biologist Dr. John Cairns. Within this paper, Kenny pointed out a quote that read:

> We are accustomed to thinking of the combination of natural variation and natural selection as a force for the good, that creates and maintains the fittest in a species and discards the unfit. This is the fundamental theorem of biology. But when we turn from the competition between the individuals of a species to the competition between the individual cells within a single animal, we see that natural selection has now become a liability.

In summary, natural selection doesn't just happen at the species level, as we typically envision it—the slowest antelope getting eaten by the lion, the male peacock with the vibrant plumage attracting a mate. It is also happening all the time, within us. Our cells compete, just as different individuals within a species do. The ones that create more copies of themselves are the victors, while those that die off or can no longer make copies have less influence shaping the subsequent generations of cells to come. But what happens when something that increases a cell's fitness is detrimental to the individual in which it resides? Cancer is one example of this. These cells are very successful from a fitness perspective. They often reproduce at a very fast rate, they take over niches in the body, and they monopolize resources. But we all know how that story usually ends—if the conquest of cancer cells is not thwarted, they become so taxing that they destroy the world around them.

Thus, when we think about aging, it does not merely come down to the robustness of each individual cell, but rather how well the system of cells and molecules synchronously work together and how that impacts the organism as a whole. Successful systems are those that are cooperative, where each cell has a specified role that it diligently carries out for the greater good. This is the root of the expression "the whole is greater than the sum of its parts." This cooperative community is the epitome of what we observe in young/healthy tissues and organs. There are different kinds of cells, each with different jobs, and they generally work together—communicating and helping each other—which leads to the success of the whole (you).

As with any good community, cells are aware of their surroundings. They receive and send signals to their neighbors, relaying information about themselves and their environment, and they call out for help or alert others when something needs to be done. This intricate cell-to-cell signaling is the backbone of how our cells are able to coordinate what seems like an insurmountably complex task of making a person starting from a single cell. During development, each cell that is made directs the actions of the subsequent cells. There are specific chronological steps based on rules encoded in our genome that are carried out in response to the signals from neighboring cells until, voilà, you have a human—at which point the process knows to stop or at least change its goals. You, or any multicellular organism for that matter, would not exist without the brilliant chemical language of cells.

As the organism ages, however, we see a breakdown of this once beautifully designed and awe-inspiring process. As cells begin to malfunction or die off, we see changes across large groups of cells, which eventually manifest as damage at the tissue or organ level. In some ways this is akin to failing societies. Like cells, people in successful societies tend to occupy specific and complementary roles. While careers may shift somewhat to meet the needs within a society, people often home in on specific domains of expertise. As a whole, the society can meet all necessary demands and the individuals can work together to ensure prosperity and stability. Another characteristic of individuals in a society are social networks. Each one of us is strongly influenced by the inputs and experiences of those around us, especially those closest to us. When our friends and family detect a threat, they let us know, and often this alters our behavior. When they experience hardship or success, so do we. We prop each other up and, in general, make each other better (or at least that is how it should be).

CELLULAR DYSTOPIA
AND THE RISE OF THE ANARCHISTS (CANCER)

So what happens to cause societies to fall apart? What factors cause chaos and break down the social fabric that made groups robust in the first place? By considering parallels in human populations or societies, we may be able to better understand the age-related demise in tissues and organs. After all, what are cells but individuals in a highly networked biological society?

Many of the things that have been implicated in the collapse of societies have parallels in biology and aging. These include overpopulation, breakdown of avenues for acquiring resources, and environmental degradation. As already discussed, the environments and infrastructure of our cellular communities are hugely compromised by the onset of age. Damaged and misfolded proteins clump together and impair cellular functioning. The structural proteins (extracellular matrix) that house our cells and facilitate communication and transmission between neighbors break down. Stressed and/or senescent cells contribute to a chronically inflamed environment that can damage neighboring cells, further propagating cell stress, senescence, and death.

In addition to the increasingly toxic environment that arises with aging, cells also experience shortages in important resources. As we age, our metabolism becomes less efficient at producing the energy needed by cells to carry out their jobs. Mitochondria, which are considered the powerhouses of a cell, decline in number, and even those that remain have accumulated such damage that it can impair their energy-creating capacity. Furthermore, our bodies also lose the ability to absorb important nutrients as we grow older, leading to lower bioavailability of critical vitamins like B12, calcium, folic acid, and iron.

As cellular environments and available resources become compromised, we also tend to see changes in the behaviors of cells. In some ways it can look very dystopian. One peculiar thing that researchers have noticed is that cells that once had specific identities and roles in young tissue tend to lose them as tissues age. It is still unclear whether this is an unintentional loss of specificity or a strategic shift. On one hand, this shift could result from the inevitable damage accumulation that is synonymous with aging. Cells may incur insults over time that rob them of the unique traits that once helped them carry out their specific roles.

On the other hand, the cells' shift away from specificity could also be a response to the deteriorating society around them. As neighboring cells die, senesce, or malfunction, the remaining cells respond to the signals being sent out by their fallen comrades. They may need to be more resilient, resourceful, and/or adaptable than they had been in the good old days, when they could still count on their social circle and work as a team. If you have ever read a dystopian novel, you know the people who survive are those who can take care of themselves—acquire food, build shelter, protect themselves, and so on. They are not the ones who are highly dependent on others. It is interesting to note that the aging cells that seem to prosper—like cancer cells—are those that can shed their strict identities and become jacks-of-all-trades. These societies don't last, though, and eventually the entire population collapses.

As I mentioned previously, a long-standing view in cancer biology is that accumulating mutations drive cancer progression and that this constant rolling of the dice explains the increase in cancer risk as we grow older. In contrast, however, a colleague of mine, Dr. James DeGregori at the University of Colorado, recently proposed what he calls the "adaptive oncogenesis model." His theory is that under the conditions observed in young, healthy tissues, normal cells prosper because they were adapted for that specific microenvironment. It is what is expected. As the microenvironment and other cellular conditions change with age, though, normal cells don't cope well. Unfortunately, the cells that can adapt to these changes and thus outperform their neighbors tend to be those that acquire cancer-related mutations—the self-sufficient, fast-growing, versatile ones. Thus Dr. DeGregori suggests that throughout life, our cells are constantly acquiring the mutations that are thought to drive cancer. It isn't until the environment changes due to aging that these cells are able to reach their potential.

AGING AS A DRIVER OF DISEASE

Up until now, a lot of the discussion in this chapter has focused on cancer, but it is not the only disease that threatens us as we grow older. As each of us moves into the later decades of our lives, we become much more vulnerable to a wide array of conditions and diagnoses that have an immense impact on our health, functioning, and overall quality of life. These major diseases of aging are believed to be the result of the molecular and cellular changes described previously. They are what emerge from the epigenetic modifications, stem cell exhaustion, telomere attrition, genomic damage, senescence accumulation, loss of proteostasis, mitochondrial dysfunction, altered cellular communication, and dysregulated nutrient sensing. In short, aging of molecules and cells is the main cause of most chronic diseases.

Cardiovascular Disease

Cardiovascular disease is the leading cause of death worldwide, killing just under 18 million people every year. The underlying roots of cardiovascular disease are strongly linked to changes that manifest with aging, and as a result, the risk of heart failure, atrial fibrillation, and/or stroke rises substantially over the life course. This is due mainly to a number of age-related changes in the vasculature and in the heart itself. As arteries age, they become stiffer as the structural proteins and extracellular matrix begin to degrade. Arteries also accumulate oxidized fatty plaques that line their walls (a process called "atherosclerosis"), protruding into the inner channel where blood flows. When cholesterol-carrying lipoproteins penetrate the arterial wall, they initiate an inflammatory response that recruits immune cells called "macrophages." Because the immune system is unable to neutralize the perceived foreign invaders, it initiates plan B, in which the macrophages will essentially engulf the lipoproteins in an attempt to create a perimeter around the perceived threat.

These lipid-laden macrophages are called "foam cells," and over time they accumulate into large, fatty streaks lining the walls or arteries. Unfortunately, as these plaques expand with aging, this in turn can restrict blood flow to tissues and organs throughout the body. If a coronary artery becomes almost completely obstructed, blood and oxygen can no longer pass through the channel, which triggers a heart attack or heart failure. Additionally, pieces of these plaques can break off due to the increasing force of blood attempting to flow through the constricted opening. When this happens, these pieces can travel along the blood stream and eventually become lodged in smaller blood vessels, often in the small blood vessels in the brain. If these pieces of plaque completely cut off blood, it will trigger an ischemic stroke. Conversely, the mounting pressure from a blocked blood vessel can also cause it to rupture and blood will seep into brain tissue, causing a hemorrhagic stroke.

Based on the etiology of both heart disease and stroke, it is no surprise that these two conditions pose risks that increase substantially with aging. Additionally, the myriad age-related arterial changes can be exacerbated by high blood pressure, which is present in almost two-thirds of adults over sixty years of age. Hypertension contributes to changes in the heart structure as well. It can cause what is called "left ventricular hypertrophy," which is an expansion in the walls of the main pumping chamber of the heart. This enlargement has the potential to compromise the elasticity of the heart muscles and may lead to a decline in pumping force, further perpetuating the age-related decline of the cardiovascular system.

Type 2 Diabetes

Type 2 diabetes is another disease whose progression is strongly rooted in the aging process. Through evolution, our bodies have developed remarkably programs to regulate the availability and storage of nutrients in our bodies. For our ancestors, this was critical for surviving the long periods of fasting-feeding that characterized their lives. At present, though, most people have the opposite problem—we have an abundance of available food, which can often result in surplus caloric intake (overeating). Overeating can disrupt the finely tuned nutrient sensing systems in our bodies, with potentially devastating consequences for our health.

When the brain detects sugar in the bloodstream following a meal, it instructs the pancreas to release a hormone called "insulin." Insulin is critical for our survival because it helps our cells take in sugar to be converted to usable energy. Unfortunately, with aging, the receptors on our cells that are meant to detect and enable insulin to enter become less responsive. When this happens, the much-needed blood sugar is not absorbed into our cells and instead remains in the bloodstream, causing widespread damage. Excess freely available sugar has the potential to cause chemical changes that damage proteins and other large molecules. This, and its co-occurrence with widespread inflammation, is partly why type 2 diabetes is an additional major risk factor for many other age-related diseases, including cardiovascular disease, cancer, and even Alzheimer's disease.

Alzheimer's Disease

Alzheimer's disease is a progressive degeneration of the brain and accounts for 60 to 80 percent of dementias. Genetically determined Alzheimer's disease—which often strikes individuals in midlife—accounts for less than 3 percent of all cases. The more common form is what is called "sporadic" or "late-onset" Alzheimer's disease, which directly results from changes that occur with aging. Generally, the risk of developing Alzheimer's disease in a given year starts increasing around age sixty-five, doubling every five years, and finally affecting nearly a third of the population age eighty-five and over. While the exact causes of Alzheimer's disease remain a mystery, scientists have identified hallmarks in the brains of people with the disease. Most of these hallmarks have to do with alterations to proteins in the brain. In general, the brains of people with Alzheimer's disease contain significant deposits of (1) plaques made up of a type of protein called "amyloid beta," and (2) neurofibrillary tangles made up of clumps of another protein called "tau." My lab and others have also found that the support cells in brains from Alzheimer's patients exhibit epigenetic patterns associated with accelerated aging.

Another recent discovery is that senescent cells may be prevalent in Alzheimer's disease. One hypothesis is that the plaques and tangles in Alzheimer's brains may induce senescence in nearby cells, in turn creating a highly inflammatory and toxic environment that causes additional damage to nearby cells. Alternatively, it may also be the case that senescent cells arise as cells age naturally and their inflammatory signatures contribute to the formation of plaques and tangles. While we are still a long way off from fully understanding what contributes to Alzheimer's disease, it is clear that the aging process plays a major role. Along those lines, it has been shown that behaviors that impact general aging also seem to strongly influence Alzheimer's susceptibility. Additionally, individuals who appear to be aging slower, like those with very strong family histories of longevity, seem to stave off Alzheimer's and other dementias for far longer than the general population.

AGING AS A DISEASE

While the risks of these diseases are associated with increasing age, it is not chronological age that determines risk, but instead biological age. Even though most of the statistics I have presented are in the context of chronological age, remember that these are all based on population averages and trends. They are generalizations. In contrast, as you think about your individual or personalized risk of disease, it is more important to assess the degree to which *your* biological profile has changed over time rather than the number of trips you have taken around the sun.

In fact, recently, there has been a push in aging research to define aging itself as a disease. The goal of this is to declare aging as something that is targetable or treatable. Not surprisingly, this is an idea that does not sit well with a great many people. Most of the criticism cites the fact that aging is natural; it is something that happens to everyone, not just a select few. Yet, in reality, both aging and the chronic conditions we so easily define as diseases (like cancer, Alzheimer's, diabetes, heart disease) are manifestations of a progressive loss of functioning in one or more physiological systems. The underlying pathologies of all these diseases also happen to everyone. Even if you do not have Alzheimer's disease, I can guarantee that some level of pathology (plaques and tangles) are present in your brain already. Same goes for heart diseases and arterial plaques, or precancerous cells. Ultimately, "disease" states are socially derived concepts. They are artificial attributes we have used to define some state. As with aging, the etiologies of all chronic diseases actually lie on a continuum. What we have done is simply to select some tipping point on that continuum and then declare that those to the left of it are "not diseased," while those to the right are. But there is nothing magical about this threshold that we have selected as a means to group people into a disease category. We simply needed a way to segregate patients because our current medical system operates from a treatment point of view, and a problem needs to be defined before you can attempt to fix it.

If we were to define aging as a disease, the same rationale should be applied. Intervening in aging is not "going against nature" any more than intervening in a disease process. What we need, however, is a way to systematically define the thing we are trying to target—a way to know whether some intervention was successful, or to determine who among us most needs a given treatment.

We need a way to actually measure aging.

4

How to Measure Biological Age

I hope by this point I have conveyed to you the importance of knowing your biological age. So, let's get down to brass tacks and discuss how one would actually go about measuring it. In truth, scientists haven't come to a consensus on the best way to estimate age. Because aging is so complex and multifaceted, there are dozens of measures that could be used. These range from things as simple as taking a selfie to multisystem assessments that require specialized technology and algorithms. In this chapter, I will present some of the ways you can estimate your biological age, many of which can even be done from the comfort of your home without the need for a doctor visit. Keep in mind, though, that there are also pros and cons to the different methods that I will discuss.

As mentioned in chapter 3, we think aging starts on the molecular level, and over time these alterations contribute to the changes that we normally associate with old age—disease, functional decline, skin wrinkling, muscle loss, declining athletic performance, abnormal laboratory results, and the like. The temporal connections among these changes have been beautifully described by one of my close colleagues, Dr. Luigi Ferrucci, who serves as the scientific director at the National Institute on Aging. In a paper that I coauthored with him and two other scientists (Dr. Pei-Lun Kuo and Dr. Eleanor Simonsick), we describe how consequences of aging at the molecular level are already observable very early in life. Yet, given the resilience of our bodies, these are not easily perceived by the individual. We are able to withstand a fair degree of damage and still seem to function with no apparent problems. But once this damage reaches a certain degree of severity, we see physiological and anatomical changes, and eventually these will reach thresholds that constrain physical and cognitive functioning.

FUNCTIONAL MEASURES OF AGING

Because aging will eventually impact all of these levels, from the molecular all the way up to the functional, information about any of these changes can be used to estimate biological age. Probably one of the simplest ways to estimate aging is at the functional level, using a measure of what we call "deficit accumulation." Aging is not just linked to an increasing immediate risk of developing *a* major chronic disease/condition; it increases the immediate risk of developing *multiple* conditions simultaneously—what we refer to as "multi-morbidity" or "comorbidity." In fact, research has shown that with every condition you develop, it takes less time for you to develop another, and this continues with each subsequent condition. The more you have, the faster they accumulate.

The deficit accumulation measure is a count of the diseases and/or high-risk conditions that a person has. One of the first examples of these measures has come to be known as "the Frailty Index." Starting in the early 2000s, a geriatrician named Dr. Kenneth Rockwood and an applied mathematician, Dr. Arnold Mitnitski, demonstrated that by estimating the proportion of potential deficits present in an individual, one could produce a fairly reliable aging estimate. They found that this measure systematically increased across a person's life span and was a good indicator of remaining life expectancy, above and beyond chronological age. Essentially, this variable was able to capture the state of a person's functional aging, which is a good indicator of vulnerability to future disease and/or death.

Another advantage of this measure is that, unlike many of the ones I will discuss later on, it is very easy to calculate, completely noninvasive, and does not require you to invest in data beyond what you may already have from your last doctor visit. There are, however, a few minor disadvantages of this measure compared to others. First, it may not be able to differentiate aging rates in younger or otherwise healthy adults for whom deficits have not started to pile up. Second, it will give you an overall biological age measure and cannot detect tissue- or organ-specific aging rates (more on this in chapter 5). Third, in estimating the number of deficits, all conditions are counted equally. We know people age differently in different systems, which may make them more or less vulnerable to distinct conditions as they age. Not all these conditions are equally deleterious for health. For instance, having a diagnosis of diabetes is more dangerous than hypertension or arthritis. Yet the deficit accumulation measures don't distinguish between the severe and the mild.

Despite these minor drawbacks, the Frailty Index is a fabulous measure for getting a quick and simple readout of your overall health and aging. In the table on the following page, I have provided a modified version of Rockwood and Mitnitski's Frailty Index for those interested in determining their deficit accumulation aging score.

Diseases	Functioning	Lab Tests
Have you ever been diagnosed with the following:	Without help or special equipment, how much difficulty do you have with the following:	At your most recent doctor visit and blood draw, did you fall within the following categories:
(give yourself 1 point for each "yes" you answer)	(score each as: 0=None, 0.5=Some, 0.75=Much, 1=Unable)	(give yourself 1 point for each "yes" you answer)
☐ Type 2 Diabetes	☐ Walking ¼ mile	☐ Triglyceride level of 150 mg/dL or more
☐ Congestive Heart Failure	☐ Walking up 10 steps	☐ HDL cholesterol level less than 40 mg/dL
☐ Coronary Heart Disease	☐ Stooping, crouching, kneeling	☐ LDL cholesterol level more than 160 mg/dL
☐ Angina	☐ Lifting/carrying 10 pounds	☐ Systolic blood pressure (top number) of 130 mm Hg or more
☐ Heart Attack	☐ Walking between rooms	
☐ Atrial Fibrillation	☐ Standing up from an armless chair	☐ Fasting glucose of 100 mg/dL or more
☐ Stroke	☐ Getting in/out of bed	☐ Albumin level less than 3.4 g/dL
☐ Cancer (count 1 for each)	☐ Holding utensils	
☐ Emphysema	☐ Standing for more than 30 minutes	
☐ Chronic Bronchitis	☐ Reaching overhead	
☐ COPD	☐ Remembering what you ate for dinner the night before	
☐ Liver Condition		
☐ Dementia		
☐ Arthritis	☐ Walking on an uneven surface without falling	
☐ Osteoporosis		
☐ Hearing Impairment		
Total Points:	Total Points:	Total Points:

Add up your points for the three categories and divide by 34. If you happen to not know the answer to all or some of the questions, add up what you do know and divide by the number you answered.

Total Score (range 0–1):
Very Fit (Score < 0.1)
Well (0.1 ≤ Score < 0.2)
Managing (0.2 ≤ Score < 0.3)
Vulnerable (0.3 ≤ Score < 0.4)
Mildly Frail (0.4 ≤ Score < 0.5)
Moderately Frail (0.5 ≤ Score < 0.6)
Severely Frail (Score ≥ 0.6)

One other drawback with deficit accumulation measures like the one presented above is that they aren't very good when it comes to helping people prevent disease or extend healthspan. For instance, they don't differentiate the health or wellness of people who have yet to develop a disease and can really only be used to track aging once diseases and conditions have started to manifest. For many people who have acquired diseases, the fact that they are biologically aging isn't a surprise. They can perceive it themselves. For seemingly healthy individuals, it is hard to self-assess where one actually stands and whether changes should be made to ensure prolonged, disease-free life expectancy. For this task, we need to quantify aging changes that precede disease diagnoses.

TELOMERE LENGTH

In the early 2000s, a new measure emerged which gave scientists hope that the quest for a way to estimate biological age was finally over. The measure was telomere length. As described in chapter 3, telomere short-ening had been identified as a major hallmark of aging. Over time, it was shown that as cells divide or encounter instances of stress and/or dam-age, the protective caps of chromosomes are shortened or degraded, po-tentially inducing programmed cell death (apoptosis) or cellular arrest (senescence). More and more cells experiencing severe telomere attrition in one or more chromosomes can contribute to cellular loss and jeopar-dize tissue integrity. Ultimately, severe telomere shortening and accom-panying cellular senescence are thought to contribute to the etiology of age-related disease and decline.

In light of this, researchers began developing a multitude of sequenc-ing and imaging techniques for estimating telomere length in anything from a few drops of blood to a whole tissue. One method, called "qPCR," showed several advantages for widespread applications. The technology required only small amounts of DNA that could easily be acquired through noninvasive procedures, and the method was generally straight-forward, not very labor intensive, and relatively inexpensive. This made measuring telomere length applicable to both clinical trials and popula-tion research in general.

In 2004, a professor of psychiatry at the University of California, San Francisco, Dr. Elissa Epel, joined forces with Dr. Elizabeth Blackburn—who in five years would go on to win the Nobel Prize in medicine for her work on telomeres and telomerase. Together, they published a ground-breaking study providing the first demonstration of the utility of telo-mere length in health research. In their paper, Epel, Blackburn, and their coauthors showed that psychological stress was associated with shorter telomere length in white blood cells, such that women experiencing the highest levels of perceived stress exhibited telomere lengths equivalent to women more than a decade their senior. The team argued that telomere attrition may be the missing biological link connecting the stress we all experience to our health and wellness.

Following the publication of this paper, most of the large epidemiological and population health studies started measuring telomere length in their subjects. The hope was that telomere length could serve as a biomarker of aging that would help researchers better understand the root causes of differences in health and disease risks across populations. Additionally, there was also optimism that such a measure could be applied to identify vulnerable groups of individuals and improve targeting of health interventions.

The year after Dr. Blackburn received her Nobel Prize, she helped found a company called Telomere Diagnostics (TDx). TDx would later offer a direct-to-consumer test to assess telomere length, called TeloYears. A few drops of blood are collected via finger prick, using a lancet similar to the ones used by diabetics to test their blood sugar. The blood spot sample is then shipped to a lab, where the telomere length is measured. The biological age that is reported back represents the average age of people with a similar telomere length. This is also meant to imply that along with their telomere profile, you may also share their health risks. But as data started to pour in on the associations between telomere length measured in white blood cells—termed "leukocyte telomere length," or LTL—the links between LTL and healthspan or life span were disappointing.

Overall, LTL appeared to exhibit fairly weak associations with age. For most groups of people, age explained less than a quarter of the variation in LTL, suggesting that LTL did not track aging very well. Moreover, there were conflicting results when it came to predicting remaining life expectancy, with some studies detecting significant associations between LTL and risk of death in a given time frame, and an equal number turning up nothing.

Eventually it became obvious that the problem with using LTL to inform our measurement or understanding of biological aging was less of a reflection of the importance of telomere biology to the aging process and more to do with how it is measured. Because of the need for efficiency and cost-effectiveness when encompassing biological measurements into large population studies on tens of thousands of people or when offering the test to consumers, one is often limited in the ability to adopt and implement the most cutting-edge and precise techniques. Thus the measures of LTL that were (and still are) being applied to these cohorts end up being unidimensional averages. What I mean by that is that every cell in your blood (except red blood cells and platelets) have two telomeres per chromosome. With twenty-three chromosome pairs (forty-six total), this equates to essentially ninety-two telomeres per cell. Using a simple finger prick method, one can usually collect 20 microliters of blood from a single droplet, which has been estimated to contain anywhere between about 100,000 to 200,000 white blood cells. That's about 10 million telomeres. As I am sure you can imagine, not all the telomeres in a sample are the same length. Some are very short and some remain long, even in older individuals. The likelihood a telomere is longer or shorter is also biased by what kind of white blood cell it is found in—telomere length is more likely to be shorter in cells that rapidly divide and replace themselves.

Unfortunately, the measures of LTL take the average across all 10 million or so telomeres in your sample. This ignores a lot of potentially insightful information. What does it mean if someone has a lot of variation in their telomere length? For instance, while two people might have similar mean telomere lengths, one could have relatively homogenous lengths across most of their telomeres, while the other person could have some very long telomeres that are counterbalanced with very short ones. Do they represent the same aging phenotype? Probably not. Another important question being overlooked is which cell types are exhibiting faster shortening—or which chromosomes, for that matter. Without these answers, telomere length measures may only give you a fuzzy picture of what is truly happening among your cells. It's unidimensional, when in reality what happens with biological aging is a multidimensional process. For this reason, measures that capture dynamic shifts across distinct yet connected systems will be much more useful for determining one's personal aging profile.

MULTISYSTEMS AGING MEASURES

In 2018, I published an aging measure that combined multidimensional information from lab tests meant to capture functioning in various physiological systems. The exciting thing about this measure was that it uses standard clinical data—things most people get measured annually during a regular checkup with their doctor. While physicians use these tests to determine if someone has an abnormal level on any one measure, there is so much more that can be gleaned from the simple printout of results, things that are all too often completely overlooked. Even if you haven't been to see your primary care physician in recent memory, for readers in the United States, the lab tests used to estimate aging are so common that they can be acquired relatively inexpensively (for about fifty dollars) by visiting either a Quest Diagnostics or Labcorp. Nearly all the lab tests used to estimate biological age are included in a standard chemistry panel and complete blood count (CBC) panels. The only measure not included is called "C-reactive protein," which can be measured using a separate test from the same blood draw.

Overall, nine measures go into the equation that together combines information on physiological states for a number of different systems, including cardiovascular, immune, liver, kidney, and metabolic, and then combines these to generate an overall biological age measure for the person. When merged with information on your chronological age, we are able to estimate what we call "phenotypic age." The term "phenotypic" can be defined as a characteristic of an individual resulting from the interaction of their genotype and the environment—and thus, we used "phenotypic age" to refer to a characteristic aging profile of an individual that is influenced by both genetic and nongenetic factors.

The nine blood measures used to estimate phenotypic age were chosen out of a panel of nearly fifty possible tests. This was done using something called "machine learning," in which a computer is programmed to develop a mathematical prediction. In this case, we were aiming to predict remaining life expectancy; thus, the combination of the nine measures and chronological age represented the best predictor of how long a person would live out of all possible combinations we considered. When independently tested, phenotypic age was able to predict who would survive the next ten years and who wouldn't, with approximately 90 percent accuracy, without having to know anything else about the person. Obviously, we couldn't predict who would get hit by a bus or who would contract some rare yet fatal disease, but the reason our measure was so accurate was that most people die of age-related diseases and we were directly estimating the biggest risk factor for death—biological aging.

For readers interested in determining their biological age from this measure, it is actually remarkably easy to do. As a first step, you would simply visit your doctor or a lab facility (like Quest Diagnostics or Labcorp) and request the nine tests shown in the table below. Once you have these results in hand, there are various freely available websites offering the equation as an online calculator. For instance, a web interface can be found at: https://www.longevityadvantage.com/mortality-score-and-phenotypic-age-calculator/. Similarly, you can download a spreadsheet from the blog of longtime lab tester Dr. Michael Lustgarten at https://michaellustgarten.com/wp-content/uploads/2020/10/DNAmPhenoAge_gen-1.xls.

Next, you simply enter in your values, and voilà, you get your phenotypic age.

Lab Test	System It Captures
Fasting Glucose	Metabolic
C-reactive Protein	Inflammatory
Albumin (Serum)	Liver, malnutrition, and inflammation
Alkaline Phosphatase (Serum)	Liver
Creatinine (Serum)	Kidney

Lab Test	System It Captures
Red Cell Distribution Width	Immune
Lymphocyte Percentage	Immune
White Blood Cell Count	Immune
Mean Corpuscular Volume	Immune

NOW WHAT?

Let's imagine you enter everything in and the biological age value that pops up on your computer screen is not what you were hoping for. The good news is, you can likely change it. A high biological age shouldn't make you feel defeated, but rather serve as a wake-up call that can help you become the healthiest version of yourself. My lab has observed a number of very interesting things—namely, that biological age is influenced by factors in your life more than by your genes.

In collaboration with various colleagues at Yale, my lab estimated the relative influence of various individual characteristics among an extremely large population of adults who were representative of the U.S. population. Our exciting finding was that what seemed to be the biggest determinant of a person's biological aging was their health behaviors. The second biggest contributor were recent stressors and adversities, followed by genetics as third. While your genes and (to some extent) the adversities you experience throughout your life are beyond your control, our study suggests the biggest influence on your aging comes down to the choices you make regarding exercise, smoking, drinking, nutrition, and sleep. This was the best news we could hope for, because it happens to be something we all have control over in our lives.

Following this study, I collaborated with my longtime colleague Dr. Valter Longo to test if we could actually reduce someone's biological age by changing their dietary behaviors. While I will discuss this study and the diet in more detail in Part II of the book, briefly, we found that people who participated in three short fasts spread out over a few months were able to significantly reduce their biological age by an average of about 2.5 years. While this may not sound like much, simulations suggested that this would hugely reduce disease burden and early mortality if participants were to partake in this habit annually (a total of fifteen moderate fast days every year).

If that is not motivation enough, we have also shown that our measure of biological aging is often reflected in your appearance. While I firmly believe that the goals of slowing aging should be to improve health, there is no denying that a great many people are motivated to slow aging for aesthetic reasons. In 2018, *InStyle* magazine published an article highlighting the astounding financial investment that the average person makes on antiaging skin creams over their lifetime. With almost a thousand products on the market, the antiaging beauty category is estimated to gross over $330 billion globally in the year 2021. Individuals who invest in low-cost drugstore products were estimated to spend nearly $12,000 over their lifetime on antiaging creams, while those with a little more cash to burn, who choose to use products in the middle-of-the-market range, averaged almost $37,000 over their lifetime. At the highest range, the crème de la crème of antiaging creams would require an investment of almost $200,000 over a lifetime. Keep in mind, these numbers don't include the spending on cosmetic procedures, like botulinum toxin therapy, microdermabrasion, chemical peels, dermal fillers, and plastic surgery. Yet what consumers fail to recognize is that when it comes to their outward aging appearance, aside from going under the knife or needle, the signs of aging are best fought from the inside out. More important, given what we have shown regarding the effects of our behaviors, one could do this without substantial monetary investment.

At the end of the day, it may be surprising that a biological age measure based on only nine lab tests can foretell something about your life span and future disease, functioning, and even facial aging. But that is just the tip of the iceberg in terms of what's possible. More recently, our lab and others have begun to estimate even more powerful aging measures using hundreds of thousands of data points. What's more, they can be collected from something as simple as a few drops of blood or even your spit.

EPIGENETIC AGE

Right about now, you might be thinking, "Hey, I've heard this pitch before!" It's true. On some level, this was the promise made by Elizabeth Holmes, as the CEO of the company Theranos— to deliver an unprecedented amount of personal health information, all from a tiny finger prick. Unfortunately, this was a false promise based on a hope rather than actual science, as was beautifully profiled by John Carreyrou in his book, *Bad Blood*. While Holmes's dream did not come true, the general idea isn't as far-fetched as it may seem. She was just looking in the wrong place. The key may lie in measurements of what is called "DNA methylation," but viewed through the lens of biological aging.

DNA methylation is an example of an epigenetic modification. If you remember, as I described before, epigenetics refers to the chemical alterations that change the conformation of your genome and regulate which parts are used or not (the recipe deciding what ingredients each cell uses to generate its phenotype). Specifically, DNA methylation refers to a chemical tag (methyl group) that is added to one of the nucleotides, or letters in the DNA sequence (A, C, G, T). Usually when we talk about DNA methylation in mammals, we are referring to methyl tags added to specific cytosines (the Cs) that lie alongside a guanine (G).

These so-called "CpGs" are scattered throughout the genome. When methyls are added to them, this will typically cause that part of the genome to fold in on itself and "turn off." The genes in that region are temporarily unreachable. When methyl groups are removed, however, the region opens back up and becomes available again. The cell is then free to use those genes to make the proteins they code for or to regulate certain processes. Because of this, DNA methylation plays an important role in a plethora of biological phenomena. It is a key regulator in development, and also can define the state of a cell—whether it is a stem cell, a differentiated (defined cell type) cell, a senescent cell, or even a cancer cell. Interestingly, it also can be used to confer something about how a cell or tissue is aging.

Studies into DNA methylation have revealed that the patterns of these chemical tags throughout your genome become substantially altered as we age. Certain sites consistently gain DNA methylation, while others lose DNA methylation. While we don't know exactly why this is (although we are starting to uncover some interesting hints), the important thing is that we have learned to decode some of these patterns, and they provide amazing insight into the health of an individual.

The profound impact of aging on the patterns of DNA methylation was first discovered in the late 1980s and early 1990s. One of the scientists working in this area at that time was Dr. Nita Ahuja, a recent graduate of Duke medical school who was completing her residency and a fellowship in surgical oncology at Johns Hopkins University. Today, Dr. Ahuja is the chair of surgery at Yale medical school—the first woman to ever assume this role—and I am also happy to call her a colleague and collaborator. Early in her career, Dr. Ahuja and others showed that the DNA methylation patterns that seemed to distinguish cancerous tissues from most normal tissues bore striking similarities to the changes observed in normal tissues with aging. This caused many to form the hypothesis that age-related changes in DNA methylation may explain why cancers become more common as we age. To put it another way, our tissues undergo DNA methylation changes that may make them more cancer-like, and thus more cancer prone.

While these discoveries were groundbreaking, it took another two decades before the first biological age measure based on DNA methylation would be developed. In 2011, a group of scientists at the University of California, Los Angeles (UCLA), published the first example of a type of measure that would later come to be known as an "epigenetic clock." That study, which was led by Dr. Eric Vilain, a UCLA professor in the departments of human genetics, pediatrics, and urology, was initially designed to identify epigenetic factors in saliva that related to sexual orientation when comparing discordant twins (where one twin identifies as heterosexual and the other as homosexual). While this didn't turn up any noteworthy clues on sexuality, the group stumbled upon the same discovery made by Dr. Ahuja and others years earlier—that age has an enormous effect on a person's DNA methylation levels. After this discovery, the aim of the project changed course and the authors set out to develop a measure that could predict someone's age based solely on the DNA methylation patterns in their saliva. It turned out to be a success. This new measure predicted age with a median error of just over five years. This means that 50 percent of all samples were predicted within five years of their actual age.

A year and a half later, in January 2013, a second Southern California group—led by Dr. Kang Zhang and Dr. Trey Ideker at the University of California, San Diego (UCSD)—developed the second DNA methylation age predictor (or epigenetic clock), this time in blood. This new clock, which would come to be known as the "Hannum clock," had a slightly lower error rate than the original clock. Additionally, the authors showed that their age predictor was highly accurate when applied to a variety of tissues and, like Dr. Ahuja has shown, was accelerated in cancer tumors.

Around the same time the Hannum clock was published, one of the

UCLA authors on the first clock paper was working on a clock that would eventually change the field of aging. After the initial finding in saliva, Dr. Steve Horvath had decided to drop everything else in his lab and pursue the study of DNA methylation changes with age. Over several months, Dr. Horvath gathered all the DNA methylation data he could, eventually compiling a database that included fifty-one different tissues and/or cell types, from over 8,000 human samples. The samples spanned the entire age range, from prenates all the way to centenarians. By applying much of the same techniques as were used by the UCSD team to develop the Hannum clock, Dr. Horvath developed a DNA methylation age predictor that could estimate age with extremely high accuracy across nearly all human tissue and cell types. The measure would come to be known as the "Horvath clock" and become synonymous with estimates of biological age.

While training for my PhD at the University of Southern California (USC) in 2014, I came across Dr. Horvath's newly published paper detailing his epigenetic clock. Just that past summer, I had published a paper that described a new biological age measure I developed using the clinical chemistry lab measures described earlier. I found it amazing, however, that a similar aging signal could be written in the molecular profile of a cell. How did this happen? What did it mean? Is it modifiable? At that moment I decided that these were questions I needed to answer. A year later, I moved across town from USC to UCLA to start a postdoc position in Dr. Steve Horvath's lab.

Over the next year, Steve and I, in collaboration with other scientists in his lab and around the world, published several papers detailing all the things the epigenetic clocks could capture. We showed that women with older epigenetic ages tended to experience menopause earlier and that surgical menopause tended to accelerate epigenetic aging. We found that epigenetic age was predictive of future risk of lung cancer, especially among smokers. Using samples from brains, we found that individuals with signs of Alzheimer's disease tended to have older epigenetic ages relative to their chronological age. With a graduate student named Austin Quach, we published a paper showing the associations between health behaviors and epigenetic aging revealing that people who ate more leafy greens, exercised, and had higher education tended to be epigenetically younger. In collaboration with another UCLA professor, Dr. Judith Carroll, we found that insomnia was linked to faster epigenetic aging. And finally, as part of a large research group that pooled together thirteen different population studies, totaling 13,089 individuals, it was shown that the relative difference between epigenetic age and chronological age was predictive of remaining life expectancy. Or more simply, those whose age was predicted to be much older than they actually were (based on DNA methylation) had a greater chance of dying than those predicted to be younger.

Yet despite these exciting findings, I was still convinced that we could build a better clock. After all, the biological age measures based on clinical lab tests that I had developed as a PhD student were stronger predictors of death and disease risk than the epigenetic clocks current at the time. Another thing that kept bothering me was that whenever I (or Steve, or anybody else) delivered presentations describing epigenetic clocks, one of the questions that would inevitably arise was, "If you use X, Y, or Z method, do you think you could get a more accurate predictor of someone's age?" The problem with this question is that they were asking if we can better approximate chronological age. What they failed to realize is that the goal of our work was to capture *biological* age. These two numbers should never be perfectly correlated when looking at a group of people, because we know some of those people will be faster agers, while others will be slower agers. If everyone's biological age perfectly matched with their chronological age, that would suggest there is no variation in the rates of aging across individuals. It also would suggest that there is no need for people to undergo costly biological tests just to give us an age we already know.

Instead, the question those people really should have been asking is,

"How do we get a better measure of true variation in the rate of aging among people who chronologically are the same age?" What is the biology that differentiates the classmate at your school reunion who is completely unrecognizable from the one who appears frozen in time? The other critical piece is to ensure that whatever variation we capture among people of the same chronological age is not just an error in our estimation, but is actually biologically informative. The supposed discrepancy between predicted age and reported age should say something about the person's future health and wellness.

Through my work on this, I came to realize that instead of predicting time since birth, perhaps what we actually wanted to predict is the relative proportion of the distance a person is between birth and death. Recall the ten-mile-long track I discussed in chapter 2. If I looked at where everyone was on that track after one hour, I would want to know what proportion of the distance they had covered. Are they crossing the finish line or only halfway? Knowing this would give us some idea of their average pace. The same goes for aging. If I look at a group of people after fifty years, some will be three-quarters of the way through life, while others may be less than halfway. This is the measure I wanted to develop using DNA methylation.

During the final year of my postdoc with Dr. Steve Horvath, I threw all my effort into developing a measure that could capture this. Looking back, I have to say that this was probably one of the most stressful times of my life. I was working exclusively from home because I was balancing work with caring for a one-year-old toddler and my terminally ill father. Because my husband and I were both on postdoc salaries, we could only afford half-day day care for our daughter in an expensive city like Los Angeles. So every morning I would drop my daughter at day care and then drive to my parents' home, which was about ten minutes away. I would then sit with my dad in his room or just outside and analyze the data for my project.

Sometimes my dad was interested in hearing about what I was doing, but a lot of the time he would just nap or sit quietly while we enjoyed each other's presence—often to the accompaniment of his favorite musician, Yo-Yo Ma (whom I still listen to today when I am working). Looking back on it now, I find it ironic that I was up to my eyeballs in data trying to create a measure that would predict the process that was taking place within my father right before my eyes. For data scientists working on problems dealing with mortality or disease, these concepts can become abstractions. But that all goes out the window when faced with them in your own life. Around midday, I would say goodbye to my parents and leave to pick up my daughter. At home, my husband and I would trade off childcare duties while we continued to work on our respective research. This went on until the summer of 2017, when I had finished the study, just ahead of my father's death and my family's cross-country move to start my job at Yale.

Two months later, we submitted the paper describing a new epigenetic clock trained to predict healthspan and life span rather than chronological age for publication. The paper, which included contributions from eighteen authors (including Steve and myself), detailed our careful integration of data from more than a dozen different studies to come up with and validate our new epigenetic clock. The core analysis involved the development of the clinically based biological age measure (using only nine lab tests) that I mentioned previously in this chapter. Because this measure strongly tracked age, but also differentiated death and disease risk among people of the same age, we built an epigenetic clock that would predict this measure instead of chronological age.

What we ended up showing was that this new clock was a much better predictor for myriad health outcomes when compared to previously developed chronological age clocks. It was strongly associated with remaining life span; tracked the number of diseases a person had accumulated; reflected differences in physical and cognitive functioning; was higher in women who underwent earlier menopause; showed acceleration in individuals with obesity and/or metabolic syndrome; captured age-related pro-inflammatory processes; suggested there was deceleration in children of supercentenarians; and was shown to be higher in individuals with HIV, Parkinson's disease, Alzheimer's disease, and/or breast cancer. Finally, perhaps the most remarkable thing to me was not that we could capture a generalized aging measure when we looked at DNA methylation in blood, but that we could use this same measure to track aging in individual tissues. For instance, using the data with which Steve Horvath originally developed his multi-tissue clock, we found that our new clock tracked age in all fifty-one tissues and cell types. Perhaps one of the most exciting of these was—saliva.

REAL-WORLD APPLICATIONS OF EPIGENETIC CLOCKS

The ability to capture an aging biomarker in saliva opens up a world of possibilities. If shown to be accurate and informative, such a measure would enable people to track their aging using a noninvasive test that could be administered in the comfort of their own home and then sent to a lab for analysis. What I didn't know was that at the time, I wasn't the only one who had come to this realization.

In October 2018, I received an email from Mark Morris, the vice president of research and development at a company called Elysium Health. Elysium Health was founded in 2014 by Eric Marcotulli (CEO) and Dan Alminana (COO) in partnership with MIT scientist and renowned aging researcher Dr. Leonard Guarente (Elysium's chief scientist). The concept for the company grew out of a discovery made by Dr. Guarente's lab during the late 1990s. While working with yeast, he and his trainees had discovered a gene called "SIR2" that, when activated, significantly extended longevity. What they later found, however, was this benefit was entirely dependent on the availability of a molecule called "nicotinamide adenine dinucleotide" (or NAD for short). Without NAD, increasing the activation of SIR2 had no appreciable effect on life span.

Over the years, additional proteins like SIR2 were discovered that together made up a family of proteins called "sirtuins." While each of the sirtuins (there are seven in humans) have different biological roles, their abilities to carry out their important jobs are all dependent on the availability of NAD. The problem is that later research started to suggest that NAD levels in blood and other various tissues decline naturally with age, leading to a reduction in the important functions of sirtuins. This led Guarente and other aging researchers on a quest to identify "NAD boosters"—molecules that could increase NAD levels and, in turn, restore the loss of sirtuin activity that accompanies aging. Elysium Health's flagship product was a supplement called "Basis," which consisted of a proprietary formulation of two essential components called "nicotinamide riboside" and "pterostilbene." Put together, this cocktail has been shown to increase NAD levels in not just mice but more recently in humans. While that is an exciting first step, what remained unclear was whether this increase in NAD translated into a slowing of the aging process.

Up until recently, the problem with human clinical trials in the aging and longevity sector was that they took forever. Imagine you're a scientist who has come up with a new potential therapy that you believe slows the aging process. You decide to recruit a group of healthy, middle-aged participants. As you are writing up your study protocol, you hit a roadblock. What outcome do you use as proof that your intervention can slow aging? If this study were in mice, you would probably use life span; but with middle-aged humans, you might not have results for another thirty or more years. What about disease? The question then becomes, do you consider all diseases of aging equally (basically your outcome would be the occurrence of any disease)? Do you look at how many diseases people accumulate? Like mortality, this may require your study to go on for decades. Assuming the benefits of your intervention are more or less immediate and are even potentially compounded over time, what you want is an estimate of aging that you could measure in real time, prior to your intervention, and then track over the length of your study. Enter biological age estimates.

This was the motivation that prompted Mark Morris to send the email to me back in October 2018. A month later, I made my way down from Yale to the Elysium headquarters in Manhattan to meet with Eric, Dan, and Lenny, and discuss a potential collaboration with the team. Elysium prides itself on being a scientifically backed company and, as such, wanted a way to provide clinical evidence demonstrating whether Basis slowed aging in humans. They knew that the answer might not be what they wanted, but they felt it was their obligation to provide their customers with a way to assess whether the product worked. What this meant was that they needed a simple at-home test that was friendly enough for the consumer, yet reliable and valid enough to serve as a biomarker of aging that could stand up to rigorous scientific inquiry. Given that I had already shown that my biological age estimate system based on methylation was a good indicator of future health and well-being, expanding on this measure was a logical place to start.

Beyond the measure I had created, DNA methylation opens up the potential to extract enormous personal insights about health and aging using a single sample. We don't have to run thousands of different tests to uncover this information. We run just one. Yet this one test provides hundreds of thousands of unique data points that can be used to elucidate a person's individualized aging profile. The other advantage of this test is that it can be done using a saliva sample, which could be collected via at-home kits similar to those employed by many of the popular genetic testing services, like 23andMe. There is no need to visit a primary care physician or book an appointment with a local lab to get a blood draw. This also eliminates issues with harmonization across labs or needing to convert units for your blood test results in order to input them onto a web page. A user can simply spit in a tube, pop it in the mail, and wait a few weeks to receive a biological age estimate.

An outstanding question remained to be addressed, however, before both Elysium and I would stand behind a direct-to-consumer biological age test based on DNA methylation. Were these tests consistently reliable at the individual level? Up until then, nearly all the studies on these measures had been done in samples with thousands of participants. When you have that many people in your study, random errors in measurement aren't a big deal—they end up washing out. But if I am going to tell an individual what their biological age is, I want that to be as accurate as possible—especially if the results could influence behavior.

Shortly after my trip to the Elysium office, I started working on data analysis to determine the reliability of my epigenetic age measure. The findings were nothing short of heartbreaking. When a single sample from a single individual was split in two and then used to measure DNA methylation levels that were then fed into my algorithm, I occasionally would get biological age estimates that were five or even seven years apart. What's more, this error seemed completely random, making it impossible to flag unless you were to measure every sample three times. With one test, you wouldn't know there was a problem, and with two, it would be impossible to figure out which of the two epigenetic age estimates was the correct one.

Not only did this present a major hurdle for using what we had created to help people monitor their own aging and improve their health, it also was a problem for using these measures in clinical trials. Remember, one of the scientific benefits of being able to measure biological age in a sample is that it will help scientists screen potential therapeutics that show promise for slowing aging, rather than needing to wait years or possibly decades to determine their effect on long-term outcomes like death and disease. If the error in such a test (which we were finding could be as much as seven years) is as big as the effect of your intervention, this would make it exceedingly difficult to determine if interventions actually slowed aging and by how much.

As I continued to look into this problem, I found that it wasn't just my epigenetic age measure that produced inconsistencies, but it was *all* epigenetic age measures. This new revelation began to erode my hopes that the science I had dedicated myself to would transcend the lab and be able to help actual people slow their own aging process and live longer, healthier lives. At the same time, I wasn't ready to give up on it, either. For months, I and the bioinformatics students in my lab tried different approaches—from applying fancy statistical techniques attempting to predict which estimates were errors in the data, to decreasing excess noise (or variation) in our data prior to calculating epigenetic age. While these attempts all minimized the discrepancy between pairs of samples, they still weren't accurate enough for me to feel confident I could stand behind the biological age estimates that I was hoping to be able to provide to people.

The answer came to me on an early morning run in the summer of 2019. It dawned on me that one of the most amazing things about epigenetic clocks is that they capture a large-scale phenomenon that is taking place in our DNA over time. They aren't just capturing changes in methylation at a few specific genes. Up until now, however, the existing clocks were based on changes in methylation at specific genomic locations (often between seventy and a few hundred). The problem, I realized, was that estimating methylation at each location is not perfectly precise, and as you add up these changes, the resulting measure ends up containing a lot of technical noise. I wondered if rather than picking a few CpGs to represent (or proxy) what was happening, we could measure the more global patterns across the genome using all the locations in our data.

As soon as this idea crossed my mind, I quickly stopped, dictated the precise steps I would take to do this into my phone (thank goodness for technology), and then sprinted my last mile home to start coding. An hour later, I plotted my preliminary results—the divided samples taken from the same individuals now matched almost perfectly. What's more, this new measure exhibited significantly stronger associations with health outcomes.

Over the following months, I worked closely with Elysium to test this new technique in their data, which included a group of eight individuals, each with nine samples taken over a few weeks. The real test was to determine whether these nine samples showed agreement in the epigenetic ages they predicted. What we discovered was that the published epigenetic clocks often exhibited large deviations ranging from two to as much as eight years, while deviations in our new measure were consistently around half a year or less. This new measure—which came to be known as "Index"—was now reliable enough to be applied in both clinical trials and used to assess biological aging in an individual, at what we call the "n=1 level."

In the fall of 2019, Index was launched as a product that allowed users to collect a saliva sample at home, ship it to the lab, and eventually receive insights into their biological aging process. While I am very proud of the measure we developed, I do want to acknowledge that I have some level of financial interest in Elysium's product. My role at Elysium is currently as a bioinformatics advisor and I have continued to work closely with the team to develop new DNA methylation–based health measures that we hope will enable people to take control of their overall health and wellness.

Despite this perceived financial interest, my main motivation for wanting measures like Index to become successful is that I recognize the power of this technology to help people. I want people to take advantage of the scientific discoveries being made in order to help them live longer, healthier, and happier lives with the ones they love: to ensure parents can be there to witness their children grow up and even grow old, partners can celebrate their love and commitment at seventieth anniversaries, and so that each of us has the time and the ability to accomplish what we set out to do in our lives.

Since launching Index in November 2019, we have continued to actively work to develop new and exciting measures and tools to provide even greater insight into personalized aging. We are still in the early phases of realizing the promise of what this technology can offer, a promise that, if achieved, could revolutionize the way we approach disease prevention and personalized health and aging.

5

The Future of Personalized Aging

The idea to measure biological age came about fifty years ago, but only recently have we acquired the data and computational resources to do so effectively. As such, the field is still in its infancy. It's true: Many of the existing biological age estimates have proven that they can capture between-person differences in health and wellness even among people with the same chronological age. They can predict future healthspan and life span with a sufficient degree of accuracy that exceeds chronological age alone. And evidence is emerging to suggest that they may be modifiable in the face of behavioral change. Yet these measures still have a lot of potential to improve if we want to harness their true power.

Until now, I have discussed biological age as a single entity or number, much like chronological age. This is how most people think of it and, in fact, even how many of the scientists studying aging think about biological age. The perception (and the way I have described it up to this point) is that each of us has a chronological age and a biological age. Biological aging is multifaceted, however, with various dimensions on which two individuals may diverge. We shouldn't assume that two people who are both chronologically thirty-six years old and receive biological age estimates of thirty-one using any of the measures mentioned previously have exactly the same biology and physiology—or even the same health risks, for that matter. No two people age the same way, and no single dimension or linear measure can truly capture the complexity of the aging process. In reality, the more facets we can reveal about someone's aging process, the better we can understand their personalized risks.

AGING PROFILES—BEYOND JUST A NUMBER

In 2020, a team at Stanford University led by Dr. Michael Snyder published a study describing aging profiles they called "ageotypes." While the concept of different domains of aging had been written about before, this study was the first focused investigation in which multiple ageotypes were measured in the same individuals and used to better define distinct profiles. Moreover, this study tracked people over time and was therefore able to determine how specific systems within a person were diverging. To accomplish this, the team undertook a remarkable data feat. They tracked over 18 million data points taken from 106 people during quarterly visits over four years. Using this data, they defined four major ageotypes—immunity, metabolism, liver, and kidney. Each subject received a score for each of these domains reflecting the levels of change since the baseline observation.

Essentially, the team was able to ask how people were diverging with age. Except this time, they were not being compared to the general population but, instead, to their former selves. What is interesting about this is, the scientists observed that the degree to which someone changed over time in each of the domains varied substantially. There wasn't a singular pattern of age-related change that fit everyone. While one subject displayed dramatic age changes in metabolic and kidney domains, with very little change observed in liver or immunity, another subject experienced very little kidney aging but more dramatic liver, immunity, and metabolic aging. The results from this study further emphasize that there is no one-size-fits-all way in which we age biologically.

My grandparents are a perfect example of this. My grandmother and grandfather were both born in the same year and survived to the ages of ninety and eighty-nine, respectively. Yet, despite having almost identical life spans, they had very different experiences in terms of not only their health and aging but also their lifestyle and the potential stressors they encountered.

My grandfather was raised by his mother and stepfather on a farm in Hastings, New York, that the family had purchased just prior to the onset of the Great Depression. He spent much of his childhood outdoors, helping with the farm animals and crops, fixing fences, and riding horses. One of his favorite pastimes was making and eating homemade fudge, which according to his diary was something he engaged in almost daily. In essence, his childhood comes across as the rendering of an idyllic life of a country boy in an early Winslow Homer painting.

My grandmother grew up in a nearby town. As the daughter of the local veterinarian, she also spent much of her time outdoors among farm animals. But around the age of ten, she developed rheumatic fever—a potentially life-threatening inflammatory complication stemming from an untreated case of strep throat. While she survived, the bacterial infection forced her to spend several weeks in the hospital followed by months of bed rest. In retrospect, this experience likely contributed to some of the conditions she would go on to develop over her life.

Following my grandfather's navy service during World War II, my grandparents married at the age of twenty-one. A year later my mother was born, followed by the births of her six siblings. Although my grandmother had a bachelor's degree in music and eventually received her master's degree (she was a very talented pianist and organist), like so

many women during the baby boom of the 1950s and 1960s, she duti-
fully occupied the role of suburban housewife. My grandfather, meanwhile, took advantage of the GI Bill available to veterans of World War II
and attended the Syracuse University College of Law. Upon passing the
bar in the state of New York, he began work as a high-powered litigator
and went on to become a senior partner at his firm and a fellow of the
Trial Lawyers Association (American Association for Justice).

At the age of sixty, once their children were grown, my grandparents
joined the flocks of other New Englanders who journeyed south for the
winter, landing in southern Florida. During that time, my grandfather
began practicing law in Florida and spent his free time on the tennis
court, basking in the southern winter sunshine. Conversely, my grandmother was already starting to experience the first signs of aging. She
developed cataracts and began to suffer from joint pain in her knees,
ankles, hips, and wrists—perhaps a lingering side effect of the rheumatic
fever she had fallen victim to as a child. In addition to cataract surgery,
my grandmother also underwent two surgeries for hip replacements and
one knee replacement. Her children joked that she was going to experience old age first, and then once she had transitioned to being the bionic
woman, could go back and enjoy middle age. Unfortunately, that didn't
happen. Nevertheless, she was determined to remain physically active
and became an avid swimmer for years. To this day, I still have vivid
memories of watching her swim down the shoreline bordering our family's cabin on Lake Ontario, waves lapping over her barely visible swimming cap.

Yet by the age of seventy-five, my grandmother experienced her first
ministroke, shortly followed by progressive cognitive and physical decline. Over the years, she found it more and more difficult to navigate the
rocky breakwater down to the lake, until eventually she was forced to
resign herself to sitting in her wheelchair atop the deck, diligently watching as her children and grandchildren swam and water-skied in her beloved lake below.

The next decade and a half was accompanied by more ministrokes and declines. My grandmother was eventually moved to an assisted living facility, progressively transitioning from low care to a high-level-care nursing home. Yet despite these major setbacks, during one of her routine physicals only a few years before her death, the doctor exclaimed that she had "the bloodwork of a nineteen-year-old in a red convertible." Truth is, she maintained the humor, sass, and sense of adventure of one as well.

My grandfather, by comparison, remained extremely healthy and active up until the year he died. He could regularly be found continuing to play tennis with friends multiple times a week. Living independently, he did all his own shopping and errands and would visit my grandmother every evening for dinner at the assisted living facility. While his bloodwork was not ideal—he had borderline diabetes—the diagnosis of kidney cancer took the entire family by surprise. Also, unlike my grandmother, my grandfather's downturn was quick—much like my father's. He spent only a few short months in a care center before his passing, which coincided with his eighty-ninth birthday. The idea that he passed away before my grandmother surprised everyone—none more than her. Exacerbated by latter stages of vascular dementia, my grandmother could never comprehend how her comparatively healthy and vivacious husband had died. Ultimately, this remained a difficult recurring realization that plagued her up until her death the following year.

THE HEALTH VERSUS SURVIVAL PARADOX

The juxtaposition of my grandparents' aging trajectories illustrates a lot of what epidemiologists and population health researchers see in the cohorts they study. In fact, these two profiles are very representative of common differences between men and women as they grow older. My grandmother experienced far more impairments with aging and had a drastically shorter healthspan but in the end attained a longer life span than my grandfather. In most countries around the world, and even in a number of animal species, females live significantly longer than their male counterparts. In the United States, the median life expectancy at birth in 2018 (which refers to the age that 50 percent of a cohort of people are expected to reach) is 76.3 for males and 81.4 for females. In Japan, males are fairly long-lived, with life expectancies of 81.1, yet this still pales in comparison to the female life expectancy of 87.5 (the longest in the world). In fact, out of 181 countries for which sex-specific data is available, there is not a single one in which men outlive women. The closest is in the Kingdom of Bhutan—a landlocked country in the eastern Himalayas, bordering Tibet. In their population of less than 1 million, life expectancies of the two sexes are within a year of each other, reaching 71.1 for males and 71.8 for females. By contrast, there are four countries, including Russia and Belarus, where female life expectancy is a decade or more longer than that of male life expectancy.

Despite the fact that, on average, women can look forward to longer lives, it's not all good news. There are a number of debilitating conditions that strike women disproportionately more than they do men. For instance, of the estimated 50 million people living with Alzheimer's disease worldwide, women outnumber men nearly 2 to 1. Women are also more likely to develop osteoarthritis and osteoporosis with age, and according to a 2000 study from the National Institute on Aging, 81 percent of women over the age of ninety experience mobility-related disabilities, whereas this same statistic for men over ninety is just 57 percent.

This discordance between life span and healthspan when comparing men and women is so pervasive that it has come to be known as "the male-female health survival paradox," or more simply either "the health survival paradox," "the morbidity mortality paradox," or "the gender paradox." Regardless of the name, it highlights a striking difference between the sexes when it comes to aging. Men die younger, but women suffer more conditions. One explanation that has been proposed comes down to the idea that because men are more likely to have lethal incidences of disease (think heart attack that kills them), they may not live long enough to allow us to accumulate data surrounding conditions of aging. In fact, our ancestors a century or so ago lived only about half as long as we do today. Prior to the discovery and widespread adoption of antibiotics and vaccines, it wasn't uncommon to die young of things like viral or bacterial infections. At the same time, conditions like heart disease, diabetes, Alzheimer's disease, and to some extent even cancer were rare events—people didn't live long enough to get them.

Of course, most males living today are not dying in their forties, fifties, or even sixties, they are living long enough to develop diseases of aging, but perhaps not so long as to accumulate a collection of diseases. Furthermore, there is evidence to suggest that those who make it to their eighties, nineties, or even one hundred or more are perhaps more biologically resilient than the ones who died at younger ages. As a thought experiment, imagine an obstacle course where each participant has to run across a beam suspended high over the water while large foam pendulums swing side to side. If you get knocked off the beam, you're out (i.e., dead). Now imagine we are comparing the success of two teams, the blue and the red. The red team tends to be made up of heavier individuals (in this hypothetical example, these are the women). Conversely, the blue team is made up of lighter individuals (which for this example represent the men). What we might see is that over time, the blue team (the men) are more likely to get knocked off the beam because they are less able to withstand the hits they take. Conversely, the red team (the women) might take the same number of hits, but are more likely to bear the brunt of the force and remain upright on the beam. As the game continues, an interesting trend emerges: The blue team is no longer enduring as many hits by the pendulum as the red team. They are making it across the beam completely unscathed. This is because the only team members left on the blue team are the fast runners who can outmaneuver the swinging obstacles (the resilient subpopulation of the original blue team).

Before the game started, we may not have been able to identify who among the blue team members would be part of the survivors even though players started with differing susceptibility to getting knocked off the beam. This idea is what demographers who study aging and mortality call "hidden heterogeneity." In essence, a population can be said to be made up of individuals with diverse levels of resilience/vulnerability. Unfortunately, these hidden differences can only be observed once mortality begins to remove the less resilient individuals. That's not to say that every individual who dies younger was more vulnerable at birth (environment and luck play a role as well), but rather that having some innate resilience will increase your odds of survival.

Back to the metaphorical game. While this selection for fast versus slow team members is happening rapidly on the blue team, the red team is experiencing much less of a transition in terms of the average speed of the remaining members. This is because even the slowest ones on the red team are better able to survive the hits. The result is that when the remaining team members are compared after a few rounds of the game, the blue team looks to have fewer bruises because the ones still in the game only made it by avoiding hits, while the red team includes players who both avoided hits and those who took the hits and persisted.

While this concept of mortality selection may have some ground when it comes to explaining some of the differences in late-life incidence of disease between the sexes, it doesn't fully account for this discrepancy. Almost everyone would agree that surviving to one hundred and beyond is an achievement only realized by the most resilient among us, regardless of sex. Yet when we look at centenarians, we find that women still experience much more disease prevalence and geriatric syndromes/impairments than men. No matter how long you wait to see the hidden heterogeneity emerge, female survivors tend to experience more deficits than their male counterparts. Overall, this could suggest that gender, whether due to differences in hormones or the impact of the extra X chromosome, may produce different phenotypes or trajectories with aging. Thus, being male or female might not only influence the rate at which you age but could also skew the way in which you grow old.

Gender is not the only defining factor that influences what your aging profile will look like over time. Behaviors, environment, genetics, and random chance also play a role in determining the path your health will take as you move through life. When thinking about my grandparents, I realize that even though they both survived about the same number of years, it becomes pretty clear that the differences between them weren't just that my grandmother experienced a steady decline that lasted decades, while my grandfather's health appeared more stable, with a sudden and unexpected decline at the end. Instead, when we look back at their changing health, we also see that they manifested very different biological and physiological profiles over their lives. The takeaway is that when we compare two people's biological aging, we shouldn't just focus on the difference in the rate of change across a single linear dimension.

FINDING YOUR OWN PATH
THROUGH THE AGING LANDSCAPE

To understand what I mean, recall the analogy of the ten-mile race that I used in chapter 2 to describe what biological aging is. I said that the point where you are in the race at a given chronological time could be used to represent your biological age. At thirty minutes, some people might be a third of the way through, while others are two-thirds of their way to the finish line. While in that example I suggested that everyone was on a single track from point A (start) to point B (finish), a more accurate representation of biological aging would be a race in which everyone starts at the top of a hill and finishes at the bottom (described in chapter 3).

The difference in this race is that there is no predefined trail. Each runner can take a different path to reach the bottom. While there are nearly an infinite number of potential paths one could take, most people will end up taking one of a handful of options to get down the hill. Yes, you could run around in a circle and zigzag back and forth, but it is highly unlikely that anyone would actually do that. The landscape or topology of the hill the runners are descending will somewhat dictate the path that they are most likely to take. Perhaps there are three general paths we can imagine most people will follow. One of these paths may be extremely direct and steep. Another a bit more gradual, with runners cutting back and forth across the face of the hill, slowing their descent. For the third, the runners may traverse a ridge slowly descending across the top of the hill, before heading more directly down a fairly steep decline.

At this point, you might be asking yourself, "What does all this have to do with biological aging?" For the original ten-mile-race metaphor that I first described, the location in the race where a runner is at a given point in time represented their biological age. It was measured as a single dimension—relative distance between birth (start) and death (end). This new race can also represent an abstraction of biological aging, but this time in four dimensions. Time is the first dimension, while the other three dimensions represent the physical location on the hill: first, the altitude or elevation or how high up you are on the hill (usually defined as Y); second, where you are relative to north and south coordinates (defined as Z); and third, where you are relative to east and west coordinates (defined as X).

This concept of modeling of how something traverses a three-dimensional landscape over time comes from the science of dynamical systems. This helps us start to think about aging as a process that involves many types of changes, in which some people may experience one type of change more than others. We don't all experience the same changes that transition us from robustness to frailty, but rather we also possess our own unique profiles of aging, and the more variables we can use to characterize a person, the better we can capture their personalized biological aging process and then use that information to predict what may lie ahead for them in the future—or better yet, how we can best intervene to change their path for the better.

In order to do this, we need to define the variables so that we can pinpoint where a given person is on the landscape at a specific point in time, and also what path they are headed down. In this example, we have three variables to define (X, Y, and Z), whereas the fourth is chronological time, which is predefined. Let's say that your elevation on the hill (Y) represents the robustness of your system against failure, or your vulnerability to death from natural causes. That's because in the way we have defined the landscape, the bottom of the hill represents the end of the race. When you are starting out, you are as high on the hill as you can be, which signifies having a very low probability of dying in the near future. It makes sense that the higher up you are on the hill at a given point in time, the less likely you are to quickly find yourself at the bottom. Basically, the probability that you will die very soon is extremely low. That's not to say it is impossible. If something unexpected came along and knocked you off your feet—like a major viral or bacterial infection or even a physical injury—you could descend very quickly. The higher the elevation you start at when the hit comes, however, the bigger it will have to be to knock you all the way down to the bottom.

This idea comes into play when thinking about something like resilience. Biological age can't predict the likelihood that you will get hit by a bus and die, but it should be able to tell us two important things about your risks. First, where you are on the hill should give us some idea of how quickly we might expect you to reach the bottom of the hill, assuming everything in your environment stayed the same. This could be thought of as your "median remaining life expectancy." Second, it also might tell us how vulnerable your position is to an unexpected external threat—something like contracting COVID-19, for instance. Your biological age (or position on the hill) might not determine whether you get COVID-19, but it might determine what would happen to you if you did.

To figure out what your position is, we also need to define the other two variables (X and Z). In actuality, we could define them using any number of things. One possibility is that X could represent the health of your immune system, while Z represents the state of your metabolic functioning. You could also define X as the number of times all your cells have divided, or your telomere length, while Z could be the efficiency of your mitochondria to convert nutrients to usable energy. In reality, we are defining the location of a person on a biological aging landscape using far more than two input variables, and as such, there are numerous potential paths people can take as they age. The important scientific questions then become (1) what determines the path each of us takes, and (2) can we jump to another path in order to slow our descent, or even climb back up the path we are on?

DO OUR GENES DICTATE OUR NATURAL PATH?

In July 2020, an experiment led by Dr. Nan Hao from the University of California, San Diego, beautifully illustrated the idea that individuals can take different paths when it comes to aging. In this case, though, these individuals were not people, but rather a model organism called *Saccharomyces cerevisiae*, more commonly known as "budding yeast." Despite being one of the simplest eukaryotic organisms, yeast share much of their biological machinery with humans and other mammals. As such, this unicellular organism has become an instrumental model for studies in molecular and cellular biology. It was also the ideal organism for the experiment that Dr. Hao and his lab undertook. The researchers were able to trap the yeast in a microfluidic device (a device that tests or manipulates liquids or gases on a microscale) so that each individual could be studied over time. By tracking two biological changes over a yeast cell's life course, the team was able to show that despite being genetically identical, the yeast tended to take one of two aging paths, which resulted in two distinct phenotypes (or ageotypes) of "old yeast."

The first "mode" or type of aging, exhibited by half the cells, involved the degradation of a part of the cell called the "nucleolus," which is the cell's factory for producing and assembling ribosomes. If you remember back to your high school biology class, ribosomes are key proteins whose job it is to make other proteins from RNA (a process called "translation"). Over time, the nucleoli in these yeast cells would become enlarged and fragmented, causing epigenetic instability in the ribosomal DNA, leading to age-related decline and eventually death.

The second distinct mode, which was displayed by the other half of the yeast cells, tended to involve mitochondrial decline due to loss of heme/iron. Recall that mitochondria are the powerhouses of the cells, and age-related declines in their number and/or function have been shown to drive aging, as cells are no longer able to efficiently convert nutrients into usable energy. While these two modes of aging were not surprising in and of themselves, what was particularly surprising about the study was that each individual yeast tended to only exhibit one of these two age-related signatures (nucleoli or mitochondrial degradation). It wasn't that they were declining in both features equally, but rather they were making an unconscious decision to maintain one feature over the other. What's more, the decision of which of these two paths to go down seemed to be determined fairly early in the yeast cell's life, such that you could look at a moderately young yeast cell and predict what phenotype it would have once it was old.

While these yeast cells were essentially genetically identical, some potentially random process was determining how each would age. But what would happen if you started out with genetically diverse yeast? Building on decades of aging research in yeast, the team generated mutant yeast strains by manipulating two genes, either SIR2 or HAP4. What they found was that these two separate mutations appeared to bias cells toward opposite aging phenotypes.

For instance, when the team deleted the SIR2 gene, about 83 percent of the yeast exhibited the first mode of aging (nucleoli destabilization). What's more, they seemed to also accelerate down this path much more than the original wild-type yeast cells that had been observed in the first experiment. Conversely, when the team deleted the HAP4 gene, nearly 90 percent of these yeast exhibited the mode 2 type of aging (low abundance of heme). As a third experiment, rather than deleting SIR2 or HAP4, the scientists forced the cells to overexpress one of these two genes. Activation of HAP4 biased cells toward mode 1 aging (95.9 percent), yet activation of SIR2 created two tendencies—it increased the likelihood of mode 2 aging (70 percent), but also led to an entirely new mode of aging that hadn't been observed in the earlier experiments. Cells occupying this third mode tended to be very long-lived and were able to moderately maintain more youthful features in both pathways (nucleoli and mitochondrial). What the results suggested was that the very large overexpression of SIR2 prevented the inhibition of HAP4, such that these yeast organisms benefited from the best of both worlds (high SIR2 and high HAP4). Basically, they didn't have to choose sides and instead experienced minimal declines in both pathways. As a final test, the scientists forced overexpression of both genes and confirmed that many of these cells displayed the new long-lived mode 3.

Overall, this beautiful experiment shows us that cellular aging can be thought of as a fate-decision process. Individual organisms determine early in their aging process which path to take—or more accurately, which systems to maintain at the expense of others. Ultimately, this determines what aging characteristics the individual will exhibit as they grow old. This also reaffirms that not everyone ages in the same way and, therefore, we need more than one dimension of biological aging that we can assess.

This becomes particularly important when considering intervention in aging. While knowing the vulnerability of each yeast to death is important in deciding what intervention one might administer, it would be more important to know which path the yeast was on—essentially, which processes need to be targeted to get the biggest benefit. As you can imagine, an intervention that boosted mitochondrial functioning would have a bigger effect on the individuals who were quickly declining in that capacity and less effect on the individuals who were already maintaining it well.

The same may be true in humans. I recently undertook a study in collaboration with my colleague Dr. Chia-Ling Kuo, from the University of Connecticut, and a team of researchers from the United States and the United Kingdom. The aim was to analyze data from nearly 400,000 people to discover genes or genetic profiles associated with accelerated aging. For this study, we considered two aging measures. Our expectation was that the two biological age measures would yield comparable results—with maybe one showing slightly stronger genetic associations. In my prior research, both measures had been shown to predict disease and mortality risk and both had been developed with the same intention to estimate human biological age. To our surprise, we found opposite results for the two measures.

One gene in particular showed the highest associations for both biological age measures, but in opposing directions, such that the common genotype (the one most people in the population have) was linked to an increase in biological age using one of the measures, but a *decrease* in biological age using the other measure. The gene was APOE (short for "apolipoprotein"). Interestingly, APOE is one of the genes most implicated in longevity and chronic disease. In humans, differences in the genetic sequence of the APOE gene leads to three different versions of the APOE protein that this gene codes for. We refer to these different versions as "e2," "e3," and "e4."

It is important to remember that for every gene, you can have two copies (one you inherit from your biological mother and the other you inherit from your biological father). So in the case of APOE, you could have two copies of the same version or two different versions of this gene. Over 60 percent of the people in the UK population (and other Western countries with similar demographics) have two copies of the common version, which is e3 (these people can be said to be e3/e3). Another segment of the population (about 25 percent) inherited the e3 from one parent and the e4 version from the other parent (e3/e4). Approximately 11 percent of the population have inherited the e3 from one parent and the e2 version from the other parent (e2/e3). Only a very small proportion of the population have no copy of e3. For instance, 1 percent of people have two copies of e2 (e2/e2), 2 percent of people have two copies of e4 (e4/e4), and 2 percent of people have one e2 and one e4 (e2/e4). If you are curious about what you have, companies like 23andMe genotype two locations in the APOE gene, which allows them to tell customers which two versions of the gene they have (e2/e2, e2/e3, e2/e4, e3/e3, e3/e4, or e4/e4).

The two rarer versions of this gene (e2 and e4) have been a constant focus of study for researchers. Substantial evidence has been found to suggest APOE genotype relates to a person's risk of developing Alzheimer's disease, cardiovascular disease, and even a shorter life expectancy. It has been estimated that people with one copy of the e4 variant have two times the risk of developing Alzheimer's disease than those with the common genotype (e3/e3). If you are among the 2 percent of the population with two copies of e4, your risk of Alzheimer's is predicted to increase nearly elevenfold. By contrast, the e2 version of the gene appears to protect against Alzheimer's disease, such that individuals with e2/e3 genotype, and especially those with the e2/e2 genotype, have the lowest risk of all.

What we found in our study was that those with two e4s were the fastest agers when we looked at the first biological age measure, but the slowest agers for the second biological age measure. Conversely, those with two copies of e2 were the slowest agers for the first biological age measure, but surprisingly were found to be the fastest agers for the second measure. When Dr. Kuo first shared the results with me, I was convinced that the only possible explanation was that we must have an error in our computer code. I asked her if she thought there was any chance the labels had been accidentally switched, because it's generally agreed upon in the genetics field that APOE e4 is overall detrimental to health—more dementia, more heart disease, and shorter life span. How could it possibly show such a strong trend toward *slower* biological aging in one of our measures? After Dr. Kuo diligently combed through all the coding and analysis, she finally convinced me that the finding was real. In fact, we looked at another data set with around 13,000 additional people and saw the same pattern.

Eventually, it dawned on me that this mirrored the concept from the study in yeast. The APOE genotype appeared to bias which type of aging individuals were preserving, perhaps at the expense of the other. We decided to take a closer look at what differed between the two biological age measures that could explain this paradox. What we found was that the measure that was accelerated for people with e4 tended to capture more of a cardiometabolic aging profile, while the other measure in which e2s showed the fastest aging was more reflective of an immune/inflammatory aging profile. When looking at other genes associated with the two measures, again we found this trend. The first was clearly accelerated in association with genes involved in lipid (fat) production and regulation, while the second was related to genes involved in immunity and inflammation.

Overall, the conclusion that people with the e4 genotype tend to have higher lipid levels and accelerated cardiometabolic aging is not surprising. APOE is a protein that helps to transport cholesterol around the body, delivering it to organs and cells that need it and/or transporting excess to the liver where it can be broken down to bile and eventually excreted as waste. The way APOE does this is by binding with other proteins and fats to form what are called "lipoproteins." You may have heard this term before in reference to low-density lipoproteins (LDLs)— what many people refer to as "the bad cholesterol"—and high-density lipoproteins (HDLs)—"the good cholesterol."

Basically, the difference between LDL and HDL is their cholesterol to protein ratio. LDL particles are large but not very dense lipoproteins made up of more than 50 percent cholesterol. In contrast, HDL (the "good form") particles are smaller but more dense. They tend to have much higher protein content and less cholesterol. Cholesterol itself is not inherently bad. In fact, it is vital to our survival. It helps form the membranes (or outer borders) of our cells and is essential for synthesizing many hormones and important substrates like vitamin D. But when we have too much cholesterol in our systems, either due to our diets or our inability to effectively clear it, we can experience negative health consequences. This includes a buildup of fatty plaques in the walls of our arteries, excess fat deposits in our livers, and even possibly increased accumulation of Alzheimer's disease–related pathology in our brains.

While we don't fully understand exactly why the e4 genotype leads to higher cholesterol and increased risk of heart and Alzheimer's disease, the leading hypothesis is that the mutation associated with e4 genotype impairs the protein's ability to securely bind to the cholesterol, which is a critical step in clearing excess from our systems. This is a theory that I am actively collaborating with my husband to study. Using computer simulations and experimental imaging techniques, we are looking at the abilities of the different APOEs (e2, e3, e4) to bind (or grab) different kinds of fat that one might find in our bodies. Figuring out what types of fats the different versions of APOE can and cannot effectively bind to might shed light on why people with the e4 genotype have more LDL floating around in their blood, clogging up their arteries and possibly contributing to the accumulation of Alzheimer's disease pathology in the brain.

An explanation for why people with e4 may have less systemic inflammation, which was the finding in my study with Dr. Kuo, is still a mystery. When we looked at the literature, we were surprised to find that we weren't the first ones to report this. A decade prior, a smaller study of around 6,000 people living throughout seven towns in the Czech Republic reported that both males and females who had the e4 version of the APOE gene had lower levels of C-reactive protein in their blood. C-reactive protein (or CRP for short) is a standard test administered by doctors to test for signs of inflammation. It usually becomes elevated during an infection and in general remains fairly low for most of us. Scientists studying aging have noticed, however, that the levels of CRP increase slightly as people age and that this has implications for their risk of developing disease in the near future.

But why would people with APOE e2, who are seemingly protected against cardiovascular disease and Alzheimer's disease, be prone to inflammation as they age, while e4s are protected against it? One possibility we considered was mortality selection. Remember the two teams who were competing to run across a beam without being knocked off by swinging pendulums? Perhaps the e2s were the strong/robust team that, despite how fast each one of them was (or how high their CRP was), they didn't get knocked off even when hit. In contrast, slow e4s (those with elevated CRP) were knocked off, such that by the time we were looking at them, only the fast ones (those with low CRP) remained. Perhaps CRP levels further compound the high lipid levels in e4s, such that those with high inflammation just don't survive. If this were true, when we compared inflammation levels in older individuals, the e4s would look like they naturally had lower levels.

Nevertheless, when we explored this possibility by comparing inflammation in a younger population of e2s and e4s, or tested whether the proportion of e4s with low inflammation increases as a function of survival, this didn't seem to account for the difference. More and more, I became convinced that perhaps genotypes like those for APOE have the ability to accelerate aging in some systems, while maintaining others. Just like what was seen in the yeast.

DECIDING YOUR PATH

If a person's genotype has the potential to bias them down one aging path or the other, is there anything that can be done to intervene? The answer is yes. Your genes are not your destiny and there is no predestination when it comes to aging. In the initial yeast study, half of the cells aged one way and the other half aged another way—despite being clones. Even when scientists deleted or enhanced the activity of a gene, it didn't completely determine the path each yeast took as it aged, it only influenced the probability of aging a certain way. Same goes for our human study. Not all people with the same APOE genotypes had similar results on the two aging measures. Rather, there was substantial variation even within groups. The difference was that the variation just tended to be shifted toward faster or slower aging depending on the genotype and the aging measure we were looking at.

The same is true for you. If you take an at-home genetic test and it says you are at increased risk of diabetes, that doesn't mean you will get diabetes. Then again, if it says you have a lower than average risk of diabetes, that doesn't mean you're home free. We are all at risk of developing a disease like diabetes as we age—and the degree to which your genes influence the probability you will develop the disease in the next one, five, or ten years pales in comparison to the effect aging has on that probability. There is also no denying that you and I started out life with slightly different biology, however, and this can absolutely impact each of our paths as we get older. It is likely the case that certain parts of you are just innately more resilient or better maintained than those same parts in me, and vice versa.

Perhaps a little less clear are advantages or disadvantages that are context dependent. In the days of our ancestors, having a robust immune system would have decreased a person's risk of dying from an infected wound or succumbing to a viral or bacterial infection. In the industrialized world that many of us live in today, though, a highly sensitive immune system could be detrimental. For the most part, vaccines and antibiotics have made it so that most of us never have to worry about dying from a major infection in our childhood or early adulthood. Yet for those of us whose immune systems are more primed to respond, this could mean our bodies may overreact to everyday stressors (things like air pollution, overnutrition, or even psychological stress), which may ultimately contribute to a chronically inflamed state that can damage our cells, tissues, and organs.

This is an example of what is called a "gene by environment interaction." The effect of a given gene variant may be context dependent. Right now, scientists are working hard to discover what environments or behaviors confer the most health benefits for a person based on their genetic profile. Unfortunately, the enormous amount of data and complex statistical modeling involved to determine this means we are still a long way off from being able to prescribe a diet or exercise regimen based on your genetic profile.

So what's the solution? We know that each of us is unique and that recommendations based on population averages and standardization may not be relevant to our own needs. The answer is to measure aging itself. Why would you need to predict what type of ager you are based on your genes, when you can actually determine that directly? The problem with genetics of complex traits is just that—they are complex. Thousands of genes likely combine to influence your susceptibility to immune aging, cognitive aging, or metabolic aging. What's more, genes aren't the only thing at play. Your behaviors, exposures, physical environment, social relationships, and even luck will interact with your genes to modulate your aging process. So rather than trying to determine where you will end up by age seventy based on factors you were endowed with at birth, we should be making those predictions based on who you are (biologically) today, compared to who you were in the recent past. Just as scientists use data to make predictions about climate or the economy, so too can we apply these methods to predict future health.

This idea isn't decades down the road, it is starting to be a reality with the technology we are inventing today. In late 2015, Dr. Michael Snyder—who led the paper on ageotypes—cofounded a biotechnology company called Q Bio along with Jeffrey Kaditz and Dr. Garry Choy. The company aims to combine information from a detailed health history questionnaire with data from vitals, whole body MRIs, and noninvasive measurements from blood, urine, and saliva samples. The information gathered during this one-and-a-half-hour appointment at their location in Redwood City, California, is then used to generate a snapshot of a person's health. As more snapshots are taken over time, customers will be able to track their changes to determine which systems are aging more or less, and at what rate. The goal of doing this is to help customers catch potential health problems before they ever arise. While the Q Bio platform can provide clients with a wealth of informative personalized measures of their health, taking a trip to California once a year to assess your aging-related biological changes may not be feasible for everyone. This is why I have also been working with Elysium Health to develop informative ways to do this from the comfort of your own home.

Elysium's first product, Index, provides a simple-to-interpret biological age measure estimated from an at-home saliva test. While this measure has been shown repeatedly to predict downstream health and wellness outcomes, it is based on population averages when it comes to epigenetic changes. Thus, this single biological age estimate puts your aging profile in the context of what is expected for the average person and may not be able to fully capture what is unique to your aging profile. To address this, I have worked with Elysium to develop a suite of system-specific aging measures that, when combined, paint a more complete picture of who an individual is and potentially where they are headed. These include measures that track immune aging, systemic inflammation, metabolic aging, cellular senescence, cognitive functioning, kidney and liver health, hormone changes, telomere length, and even DNA damage. The amazing thing is that so far it seems that these can all be approximated from your pattern of DNA methylation in saliva. A simple test that a person can administer themselves can be used to unlock a wealth of information about that individual's aging profile, their future health outlook, and, we hope, the best prescription for improving their overall well-being. What's more, by continuously tracking these measures, we will be able to move away from comparisons between an individual and the population average. In reality, the best reference point for determining how you are aging is not the average person your age, but rather your younger self.

Finally, probably the most important reason to track changes in all these systems is to help take back some control over your aging process. Yes, aging itself is inevitable (at least for now). But that doesn't mean the way you age is already set in stone. You have some say in what path you take. By first discovering which path you are on and how fast you are going, you may be able to change course by discovering which behaviors or factors in your life you can alter in order to optimize your health and slow your biological aging process.

Part II

TAKING CONTROL

Part II

n the summer of 2019, while attending a scientific aging and longevity meeting in New York City, I was introduced to Peter Ward and Michael Geer. Ward and Geer were serial entrepreneurs who had proven they could achieve amazing success developing consumer subscription businesses for hundreds of millions of users. Now the two had their sights set on an even more ambitious venture—to develop a platform to help customers measure and track their aging process. The focus of their start-up, Humanity Inc., was less about developing new technologies to measure biological aging and more about the power of optimization. In our meeting, they described a future where everyone would routinely measure their aging process and use it as feedback to inform what they do in their everyday life. Much the way an athlete tracks their heart rate to improve their athletic potential, so too could we track biological aging to improve health and well-being. Yet, when it comes to athletics, individuals have spent decades discovering how to best improve performance. When it comes to aging, we still have a lot to learn.

BIOLOGICAL AGING MEASURES
AS A GUIDE TO HEALTH OPTIMIZATION

In recent years, the number of biotechnology companies focused on tackling biological aging has exploded. What's more, the space is starting to be occupied by real science. Gone are the days when aging and longevity therapeutics were synonymous with snake oil and magic elixirs pedaled by opportunists looking to make a buck off people's fear of mortality. While charlatans certainly still exist, the potential benefits of investment in aging and longevity is starting to spark interest from real players. Companies are recognizing the large-scale impact aging has on health, as well as the universality of the process. In response, big names are betting big money that aging can in fact be slowed—and in a manner that will produce a large increase in human life span and healthspan.

In 2013, Google (now restructured as Alphabet Inc.) founded the California Life Company, also known as Calico. The company hired a slew of famous biologists and geneticists, including famed aging researcher Cynthia Kenyon. Under the guidance of its CEO, Arthur Levinson, it set out to discover the secrets to "health, well-being, and longevity." Similarly, that same year the esteemed scientist Craig Venter, who was an instrumental player in the mapping of the first human genome, partnered with Peter Diamandis—founder of XPrize and cofounder of Singularity University—to launch the company Human Longevity Inc. The goal was to compile an immense database of human genotypes and phenotypes which could be mined using state-of-the-art informatics to discover ways to fight aging. While revolutionary therapeutics that target aging have yet to hit the market, many are confidently stating that a major breakthrough is on the horizon, aided by the hundreds of companies and university laboratories who have made it their mission to discover an authentic "fountain of youth."

Since the inception of the powerhouse companies like Calico and

Human Longevity nearly a decade ago, the industry has continued to expand. In a December 2019 contribution to *Forbes*, journalist Margaretta Colangelo wrote, "The Longevity industry will dwarf all other industries in both size and market capitalization, reshape the global financial system, and disrupt the business models of pension funds, insurance companies, investment banks, and entire national economies." This investment, both financially and intellectually, from some of the biggest companies in the world has boosted optimism in the belief that humans will actually be able to intervene in our own aging process. While some have gone as far as to suggest we may actually "solve death," most of us are focused on helping people increase their healthspan, perhaps gaining just a decade more of healthy, disease-free life.

Unfortunately, one thing that may be slowing scientific progress in the field is a lack of conceptualization of what these companies are actually trying to target. The major biotechs focused on aging and longevity all have a similar goal, which is to slow aging and improve health and well-being. Doing so, however, will depend on our ability to define aging, health, or well-being. How will we know if a therapeutic is successful if we can't actually measure the outcomes we are hoping to target in the first place?

For decades, due to the lack of reliable and valid measures for quantifying aging, most of what we have learned over the years when it comes to slowing aging has stemmed from discoveries based in other organisms, namely yeast, worms, flies, mice, and so on. Because these animals don't live nearly as long as humans, quantifiable measures like life span could be used to represent or proxy biological aging. In fact, more than a century ago, scientists started conducting what are called "life span experiments," in which they would manipulate the diets and environments of these model organisms to see if they can make them live longer. When successful, the conclusion was that the intervention being studied must have slowed the animals' aging process.

This is how most of the regimens, supplements, and drugs that I will cover were first identified as potential interventions of aging. The problem is, we know from drug studies in other realms like cancer and Alzheimer's disease that what works for a mouse won't necessarily work for a human. What's more, most of these experiments were conducted by keeping everything else as constant as possible. The animals are all almost genetically identical and housed under exactly the same conditions. Traditionally, all are male, and only recently have researchers started to make an effort to use male and female animals and actually test the effect of sex.

TESTING AGING INTERVENTIONS IN HUMANS

While animal models can point us in the right direction of what might work to slow our aging, especially as we expand our studies to include more diverse genotypes and demographic and/or environmental characteristics, what we really need are scientific findings from humans. Yet, in addition to the fact that humans are inherently more genetically and behaviorally diverse, the other problem with discovering aging interventions in humans is that the measures like life span that we have relied on for centuries to proxy aging aren't feasible. Humans live far too long. For instance, to do a life span experiment in humans, one would either have to start an intervention trial in older individuals (say those ages eighty and over) or concede to a multiple-decades-long trial that could even outlive the researchers who initiated it.

The solution: measures of biological age. Assuming we can use real-time biological data to accurately assess the extent of aging in a person, tissue, or even a cell, one could test the impact of interventions and behaviors at any point, ultimately compressing the time needed to run a clinical trial from decades to years or even months. In fact, discussions have begun with the U.S. Food and Drug Administration (FDA) to permit biological age measures to serve as evidence when it comes to approving drugs that specifically target aging, rather than a disease, outcome.

Unfortunately, our own aging doesn't stop while we wait for scientists to discover the secrets to health and longevity or for the FDA to determine whether aging is an outcome they will consider approvals for. So while we bide our time waiting for science to come up with a solution to slow aging down, another important question then becomes, What power do we already have now to intervene? In truth, there is actually a lot most of us can be doing right now on our own to improve our health and well-being when it comes to aging. We don't need to sit around hoping and praying for a eureka moment to come out of one of the thousands of labs worldwide studying the biology of aging. We can make everyday changes that may even have as big an effect as any approved drug that hits the market in the coming years. The key is to figure out what actions to take. Which changes in your life will get you the most bang for your buck? The only way to do this is by tracking your aging.

WHERE DO WE START?

Going back to the example of athletic performance, much of the advice athletes currently operate under wasn't necessarily discovered in a lab. In reality, much of it came down to things learned by the athletes and their coaches through trial and error. Incremental adjustments would be made to a training regimen, fine-tuning every action to decipher what worked. If a change worsened performance, athletes would go back to doing what they were doing before, or try something else. Growing up, I remember playing a game in which one friend would close their eyes and start moving around a room. The rest of us would yell "warmer" if they were approaching us, or "colder" if they were going in the wrong direction. For athletes, the idea of warmer versus colder can be easily assessed. It is synonymous with their performance in their given sport. We can measure if a runner's pace is faster today than it was last month, if a golfer's score improved over their prior tournament, if a tennis player has increased the velocity of their serve, or whether a baseball player's batting average is increasing or decreasing. But when it comes to aging, how do we know if we are headed in the right direction?

Up until recently, there was very little information we could use to determine this because, prior to a few years ago, we had no way of measuring biological aging with high validity and reliability. We had no way to determine whether what we were doing in our day-to-day was having an impact, be it positive or negative. Of course, we have all heard people tout the benefits of some regimen or other. It may make them feel energized or see a younger version of themselves in the mirror, but what we needed was a way to distinguish placebo (or subjective) benefits from true, objective benefits. What was the actual decrease in biological age for a person who started eating a ketogenic diet? What's the impact of the daily strolls you started taking with your friends? Is that new/popular supplement really working? Is your travel and work schedule actually "killing" you?

The power of biological age measures is that they help us answer these types of questions. Just like figuring out how to get your mile time down, so too can we test for ourselves how to slow our aging. As a disclaimer, I am not in any way suggesting that people go out and start randomly experimenting on themselves. Instead, we can build off what we already know. For instance, most of us have a general idea of what a healthy diet is in comparison to an unhealthy one. I don't think anyone will argue that three courses of fried or sugary food every day is ideal. Instead, we all have a concept that whole, unprocessed foods are beneficial for our health. But there can still be variation when it comes to the exact composition of an ideal diet. The same is true for exercise. We should all be trying to partake in it, but how much and what kind of exercise is best for our health remains an open question. Sleep—too little and too much is detrimental, but what is optimal, and is quality more important than quantity? Stress—some is beneficial, but most isn't. How do we distinguish? This is where biological age tracking comes in.

Luckily, there is a lot we already know from studies in animals or from the epidemiological research observing human populations. In part II, I will describe where that science stands when it comes to things like diet, exercise, sleep, and psychosocial stress. Again, there currently is no single definitive answer, but rather general guidelines. Right now, these guidelines can be used as a starting point from which small changes can be made to help determine what works for a person and what doesn't. It is what I like to call the "DIY approach to optimizing aging."

However, the trial-and-error approach may also not be optimal. Say we are measuring our aging once or twice a year (as is currently recommended). How long would it take to settle on the optimal routine? Moreover, with so many variables in our lives that could be altered—diet, exercise, sleep, stress, et cetera—how do we disentangle the impact of each one? Is biological age tracking something that should be treated in the same way one would do an elimination diet to discover a food allergy—that is, focus on one component at a time until you discover the right combination?

As of now, the current state of age tracking is focused on the trial-and-error approach. But additional help is on the horizon. Scientists, including myself, are working diligently to develop ways to predict how best to slow biological aging for a given person. If we are successful, the aging measures of the future will not only provide individuals a glimpse into how they are doing at the moment, but also provide concrete guidance for what they should be doing to improve.

In moving forward, we hope to harness the power of machine learning and artificial intelligence to predict the impact of behaviors on an individual's biological aging process. When I met with Peter Ward and

Michael Geer of Humanity Inc. in New York City in 2019, they described this as something akin to a Waze app for aging. Waze is an application owned by Google that provides turn-by-turn navigation based on prior input from other users. By collecting anonymous GPS locations, speeds, accident reports, and traffic jam encounters from users, it can learn and recommend the most efficient and time-saving routing and traffic updates. The ability of the algorithm to optimize directions depends on the accuracy and amount of data it receives from its users. Another example of this is Spotify, the Swedish digital music streaming service. By comparing a user's song playlists and listening habits with those from the billions of other playlists created through the service, the algorithm underlying the platform can learn an individual's preferences and use that to make recommendations.

Currently we are working to make this same idea possible for the health and aging applications of the future. As more and more people continuously track their biological aging while simultaneously reporting back what they do in their everyday lives, algorithms can begin to learn what actions produce the biggest effects for people like you. While we aren't there yet, the recent introduction of biological age products into consumer markets is a start in growing the anonymized database needed for training computers to make these kinds of predictions for current and future users.

Finally, before we jump into discussions of associations between various health behaviors and aging, I want to briefly touch upon an important concept for you to keep in mind when reading this section of the book. Scientific knowledge is dynamic. Science is a never-ending quest to discover the truth about our world, and thus that understanding of the world is ever-evolving. While this is a concept that most scientists accept without hesitation, it is also something that becomes particularly frustrating to the general public, which often looks to science for advice on what to do in their personal lives. In fact, this uncertainty is often used to sow seeds of doubt when it comes to scientific and health advice.

It is true that in the past we have touted a particular diet as the best for our health, only to find a decade later that advice changes, sometimes even 180 degrees. Likely some of what I write about in this book will be contested as we continue to learn more in the years to come. The way to minimize these about-faces, however, is to amass a wealth of informative and reliable data. Any statistician will tell you that more data usually lead to better accuracy, or an increased likelihood that our assertions actually match the truth. For this reason, continuously tracking biological age can do more than improve your health; it may also serve to extend longevity of future generations.

6

Eat (Less) to Live

Those that feed on flesh are brave and daring but are cruel. Those that feed on *qi* [attain] illumination and are long-lived. Those that feed on grain are knowledgeable and clever but short-lived. Those that do not feed on anything do not die and are spirits.

—*The Huainanzi*, 139 BC

Undoubtedly, some of the most successful lifestyle interventions aimed at manipulating the pace of aging and extending healthy longevity have been nutritional. As far back as 450 to 350 BC, the "Father of Medicine," Hippocrates, routinely drew links between health and nutritional quality and quantity. In fact, the English word "diet" comes from the Greek word *diaita*, meaning "manner of living." Throughout his thousands of pages of writings, Hippocrates extensively cautioned about the impact one's diet may have on disease risk. In an excerpt from *Aphorisms* of the Hippocratic Corpus, he suggested that nutritional excess could contribute to early mortality, stating, "Old men have little warmth and they need little food which produces warmth; too much only extinguishes the warmth they have." Additionally, he offered up advice on proper caloric intake, the correct timing of meals, and the balancing of dietary factors (although mostly in the context of the four humors theory).

THE SCIENTIFIC FOUNDATION FOR CALORIC RESTRICTION

While many ancient civilizations, including the Greeks, Romans, and Egyptians, touted the potential health benefits of caloric reduction and fasting, it wasn't until the eighteenth century that their impact became the focus of scientific study. In 1909, the Italian scientist Dr. Carlo Moreschi was the first to show that the reduction of caloric intake could slow or even stop the growth of tumors transplanted into a mouse. Five years later, this observation was confirmed in a study by Dr. Peyton Rous—the famed American cancer researcher who would go on to win the Nobel Prize in medicine in 1966 for his discovery of a cancer-causing virus. In his manuscript published in 1914, Rous suggests that "it is conceivable that recurrences of certain human tumors and the development of metastases may be delayed or prevented for a period by methods somewhat similar to those employed against spontaneous mouse tumors in the present investigation." Basically, he was proposing that caloric restriction (CR) could prevent or delay cancer recurrence and metastasis. The idea that it could also extend life span wasn't far behind.

In 1917, a team of researchers noticed that female rats whose growth had been nutritionally stunted appeared to live much longer than their normally fed counterparts. The team had not set up to study the life span effects of nutritional intake. It came about somewhat by chance. The group had been conducting numerous nutritional studies in rodents as part of their work at one of the preeminent scientific institutions of its time, the Sheffield Scientific School in New Haven. While no longer around today, the Sheffield Scientific School was a college founded in 1846 in what is now the oldest dormitory at Yale University—just a short walk from my office. Prior to being officially incorporated as part of Yale in 1945, the "Sheff School" became known as the first school to simultaneously incorporate the sciences and liberal arts into its curriculum. It produced an impressive roster of esteemed alumni and was home to a number of notable faculty, such as Josiah Gibbs (the American physicist) and Lafayette Mendel (the discoverer of vitamins A and B). In fact, it was Mendel who, while at the Scheff School, joined forces with two other remarkable yet lesser known scientists from the nearby Connecticut Agricultural Experiment Station—Thomas Osborne and Edna Ferry—providing the first ever empirical evidence for the potential longevity effects of CR.

Edna Ferry was the daughter of the civil engineer Charles Addison Ferry, who designed the famed Yale Bowl. After graduating from Mount Holyoke College, she entered Yale Graduate School, and in 1913 became the first woman to receive a master's of science degree in physiological chemistry from Yale. After finishing her degree, she worked as a scientist at the Connecticut Agricultural Experiment Station, where she met Osborne. According to her obituary, she was considered "one of the most promising of the younger women engaged in the field of biological work," up until her death in 1919 at the age of only thirty-six—just two years after the publication of the team's observations on CR.

Thomas Osborne (who served as the lead scientist on what would become a groundbreaking paper) attended Yale as an undergraduate before continuing on, receiving a doctoral degree in chemistry. Upon graduation, Osborne began working at the Connecticut Agricultural Experiment Station in 1886. In 1909, he began a collaboration with Lafayette Mendel, which enabled the discovery of CR and longevity. Working together, the two men were able to develop a novel technique that allowed them to measure the precise nutrient intake of the rats they were studying. This led to the discovery that two amino acids (tryptophan and lysine) are essential amino acids (meaning the body can't produce these amino acids on its own, therefore they need to come from the diet of the animal). As a follow-up, they also showed that they could control the growth rates of rodents by altering the levels of lysine in their diets. Low levels of lysine could stunt growth; growth, however, could be initiated again at later ages by the introduction of lysine in the diet. This technique also eventually led to the discovery of vitamin A through comparisons of growth and survival rates of rats fed diets containing dried whole milk or its various constituents, such as lactose, salts, and lard. Yet it was through their various growth experiments studying the effects of various diets, including high-protein, low-carbohydrate, and low-fat diets, that they started to notice the long-term effects of CR on life spans.

The results Osborne, Ferry, and Mendel published in 1917 were observational and had not been part of a rigorous experiment to test the impact of diet on longevity. In fact, it took another eighteen years for someone else to take up the torch.

In 1935, Clive McCay, an American biochemist, worked with two leading animal nutritionists at Cornell University, Mary Crowell and Leonard Maynard, to experimentally demonstrate the longevity impact of CR. Using rats, the team showed that reducing calories below standard levels actually extended both the median and maximal life span of the animals. What this meant was that the majority of calorically restricted animals survived longer than the majority of those kept on a control diet, and, moreover, the maximum age achieved by the longest-living animal in the group was older for the group eating less versus those kept on a normal (not excessive) diet.

Although initially dismissed, this groundbreaking study confirmed the findings from Osborne, Mendel, and Ferry, laying the groundwork for research into dietary studies on longevity. Today, the practice of CR is seen as the archetypal lifestyle intervention in the aging field. By the year 2020, more than six thousand papers citing CR's longevity effects had been published. Many of these papers, documenting how a diet comprising a reduction in calories without malnutrition (typically a reduction of 30 to 75 percent) can extend the median and maximal life spans of various organisms, including worms, flies, yeast, and rodents. Additionally, numerous studies suggested that CR not only helps animals live longer, but also helps them stay healthier, as more recent experiments have begun providing evidence that CR often contributes to an extension in healthspan by delaying the onset of various age-related conditions and diseases.

ENERGY AND AGING

While the results in animals are irrefutable, the question remains: Why does a major reduction in food intake seem to slow the rate of decline with age? At first, this seems like a paradoxical phenomenon given that the way living systems are able to actively prevent or delay the inevitable accumulation of damage is through the use of energy to repair and maintain. And for animals, the single source of energy is food. Thus, one might think that more food should equate to more energy, and more energy should signify great system maintenance. That might be true if (1) our bodies were perfectly efficient energy factories, and (2) were optimized to allocate all additional resources toward maintenance. Yet, in reality, no system or machine is perfectly efficient, and we were also not initially designed to need to maintain ourselves much past a century.

Ultimately, there is a top limit, or ceiling effect, to the amount of usable energy that our bodies will generate (what we think of as our metabolism). If our dietary intake exceeds that, the excess is then stored in skeletal muscle (for local needs) or in liver or fat cells so that it can be used in times when food is scarce. This is a beautiful system that kept our ancestors alive, but it can also be inefficient in many ways. Breaking down, converting, storing, and rereleasing nutrients costs energy, and what's more, it contributes to damage accumulation. Yet with CR, we utilize this system much less. Assuming minimum energy/nutrient needs are being met, doing so should have a positive effect by reducing excess biochemical processes and thus minimizing damage and dysregulation.

The other important part of this balance has to do with energy utilization. Ideally, we would want energy to only be used to do the most important things. What we might consider those things to be in terms of longevity and healthspan promotion, however, may be different from what our bodies have evolved to prioritize in order to maximize evolutionary fitness. For instance, in an unsafe environment with lots of predators, growing a large body mass and having constant energy stores in muscles to enable immediate activation of a fight-or-flight response is critical to survival. But will that slow aging? Probably not. Similarly, species living in constantly changing environments will need to be more adaptive/reactive, but again, that heightened reactivity may actually accelerate the aging process.

Scientists have hypothesized that CR may initiate a program that purposefully shifts energy utilization away from some things in promotion of others. Basically, your system goes into power-saving mode by turning off (or at least turning down) processes that may be less critical to surviving a period of food scarcity. Your body is hunkering down, taking care of what it has, and waiting for a more prosperous time when it will once again be able to turn all the lights back on. In the case of long-term CR, that day never comes and instead your body maintains this reoptimized state in which you are both generating less damage (because you are doing less), but also prioritizing system stability and integrity over things like growth and responsiveness. Your body is going with the defensive rather than the offensive strategy.

Trying to determine the exact mechanism through which CR contributes to longer lives and less disease will also help address another critical question: Does it work in humans? While this has proven somewhat difficult to test directly, around the world a small group of people were willing to take that bet. In 1994, a group called the Calorie Restriction Society began to take form. The creators—Roy Walford, Lisa Walford, and CR Society president Brian M. Delaney—introduced the CRON-diet (Calorie Restriction with Optimal Nutrition), hoping to attract a following of CR enthusiasts (known to some as CRONies). They defined calorie restriction as "the consumption of a diet with adequate quantities of all essential nutrients, except that the energy content of the diet (caloric intake) is safely reduced (by as much as 10 to 40 percent) below the amount of energy (calories) that the body would tend to naturally desire, absent any special dietary measures." This would mean that the average man would consume approximately 1,200 to 2,400 calories a day and the average woman between 1,000 and 1,800 per day. The reason the group was confident that such a routine would improve health was because Dr. Roy Walford had recently been a guinea pig in a somewhat accidental experiment that showed just that. It was called Biosphere 2.

THE ACCIDENTAL HUMAN EXPERIMENT

Like something out of a scene of *The X-Files*, the glass and steel domes of the Biosphere 2 research facility create a striking juxtaposition to its desert backdrop of southern Arizona. Constructed in the late 1980s, the 3.14-acre facility remains the largest closed system ever built, designed as a miniature version of what is known as Biosphere 1 (aka Planet Earth). It comprises multiple distinct biome areas, the largest of which is a 27,000-square-foot agricultural system and human habitat. To the east of these living spaces, scientific laboratories, and expansive farming quarters lie various mini-ecosystems, including the 20,000-square-foot rainforest with a 25-foot waterfall; a 9,100-square-foot ocean, complete with coral reef; a 14,000-square-foot savannah grasslands; a 4,800-square-foot wetlands; and a 15,000-square-foot fog desert. Lastly, accessed only through the system's underground tunnels, is an enormous circular chamber called "the lungs." This engineering marvel was designed so that the galvanized roof of "the lungs" could expand (actually breathe) in order to offset the change in air density as the blistering Arizona sun heated up the air inside Biosphere 2.

While some small scientific studies are still conducted within the enclosed structure, the groundbreaking experiment it was initially designed for commenced on September 26, 1991.

On that early summer morning, the world watched as eight brave scientists entered the large dome and the airlock was sealed behind them. The plan was for the Biospherians to spend the next two years sealed from the outside world to test whether an entirely closed and self-sustainable ecological system could potentially support human life in outer space. The recycled water, oxygen, and food would all come from inside the facility, with nothing but solar power being generated from beyond the glass ceiling. The international team was made up of four men and four women, among them Dr. Roy Walford, who served as the group's chief medical officer.

Walford was a physician and professor of pathology at UCLA who studied the effects of CR in mice, and showed experimentally (like McCay had) that life span could be increased by upward of 50 percent in rodents fed restricted diets. Upon entering Biosphere 2, Walford was soon presented with a natural experiment for studying this phenomenon in humans. Approximately three thousand plant and animal species were housed within Biosphere 2, which had to serve as all the components of the diets of the eight crew members for the two years in which the doors to the outside were supposed to be sealed. Having no prior agriculture experience among them, the Biospherians worked together to farm crops, raise and slaughter livestock, and prepare meals. Unfortunately, the task proved harder than anticipated and Biospherians had to sustain themselves on extremely low quantities of food.

It was estimated that prior to stepping into the mini-world of Biosphere 2, the scientists had averaged approximately 2,500 kcal per person/day. Over the first six months, though, the team members reduced their consumption down to only 1,784 kcal/day, despite the intense physical labor each was performing—including spending about a quarter of their waking hours tending to animals and crops in order to ensure their next meal. Over the span of eight months, the majority of the crew had lost about one-fifth of their body weight. In a 2018 article in Dartmouth's *Alumni* magazine, one of the Biospherians, Mark Nelson, reflected that "hunger became a new experience—and our constant companion." Nevertheless, while energy intake was extremely low, Walford remarked that the mostly plant-based diet (with occasional dairy, eggs, meat, and fish) that he and his fellow comrades consumed during their time in Biosphere 2 provided superb "nutrient density."

While a number of things went awry under the glass views of the Arizona skies—including loss of oxygen levels, social riffs, and die-off of pollinating insects—one thing seemed to be a clear success. Despite loathing the pangs of hunger they lived with for two years, the team emerged from Biosphere 2 on September 26, 1993, in what seemed like remarkably good health. In addition to fat loss (reaching levels analogous to elite athletes), the crew also experienced remarkable drops in blood pressure, cholesterol levels, and glucose levels. Unfortunately, for most of the participants these improvements in health were short-lived and the majority returned to initial levels within two years of the experiment's end.

Today, it is hard to say whether the CR brought on by their time in Biosphere 2 will result in any gains in life expectancy for the crew. So far, all the team members except Dr. Roy Walford are alive and healthy. Dr. Walford unfortunately died in April 2004 of complications from amyotrophic lateral sclerosis (ALS), just short of his eightieth birthday. One way to get at this question could be to compare the biological ages or health status of the crew to those in the general public, but this comparison is not entirely fair. For one thing, the crew of Biospherians are not a random subset of the population that they came from. Instead, they have uniquely defining characteristics, which is why they were part of the team in the first place. They are all highly educated scientists, many are doctors or ecologists, and thus occupy a certain socioeconomic strata in society. They also report having similar lifestyle priorities, mostly in terms of being environmentally and health conscious. While there is equal gender distribution, no racial or ethnic minorities were included in the group. This presents a challenge when trying to determine who in the general population they could be compared to.

Herein lies the crux to most human nutritional studies. The vast majority are not what we call "randomized control trials," where subjects are assigned to either an intervention group or a control group at random, thus removing some systematic bias. Instead, most of the time people self-select into a group. They decide to eat a certain way (e.g., plant-based, Paleo, traditional Western diet), and what usually drives them to do so are their behavioral, lifestyle, and demographic characteristics. In the case of the Biospherians, they may not have selected to undergo CR, but they did volunteer to spend two years inside a three-acre structure with seven other people, completely cut off from the outside world. There was no Biosphere 3 in which another group was randomly assigned to and supplied with ample calories as a control.

The question of whether humans can expect the same benefits from CR as are seen in animals is a critical one, and scientists have not given up trying to answer it. As a first step, they looked to our close relatives, nonhuman primates. The benefit of studying nonhuman primates over mice or other animal models is because humans are closely related to them in terms of evolutionary history. We share many of the same genetic, physiological, and even behavioral characteristics. The other advantage, in comparison to studying humans directly, is that the conditions of the experiment and the diversity of the populations being studied can be tightly controlled, making the group receiving the intervention comparable to the control group on all other fronts. They live in the same environment, share similar genetics, have similar experiences, and so on.

That isn't possible in human studies. We all have very diverse lifestyles and experiences beyond whatever the experimental condition might be, and these variations could make it hard for researchers to determine the impact of an intervention like CR, when so many other factors might be altering the outcome they are studying. The other, and possibly most important, advantage of using nonhuman primates versus humans is that the scientists know exactly how much each animal is eating. When you tell participants in a study to start on a calorie restriction diet, there are only so many tools you have to actually make sure they are following the experimental protocol. All too often, natural instincts, social pressure, and even everyday stressors can all override even the most obedient participant's sense of duty to the science. Like the Biospherians, however, the monkeys put on the diet had no say in the matter, and may be able to answer whether launching a full-on clinical trial of CR in humans would be worth the challenge.

HUNGRY MONKEYS

In the late 1980s, two consecutive trials of calorie restriction had been initiated using rhesus monkeys—one at the National Institute on Aging

(NIA) in Baltimore, Maryland, and the other at the University of Wisconsin, Madison (UW). After about two decades of meticulous research involving constant regulation of the diets, detailed reports of body weight and physiological parameters, and tracking of deaths, the results were finally in for the study from UW. As the title of the article published in *Science* in 2009 suggested, it appeared that "CR Delays Disease Onset and Mortality in Rhesus Monkeys." Eureka! The authors reported that 80 percent of their calorically restricted monkeys were still alive at the time of publication, compared to only 50 percent of the control monkeys. What's more, not only were the calorically restricted monkeys still alive, but they appeared significantly healthier. This group exhibited substantial reductions in incidence of cardiovascular disease, cancer, diabetes, and even showed signs of slower brain atrophy with age. Following publication of the study, the *New York Times* published an article in 2009 declaring that the "long-awaited study of aging in rhesus monkeys suggests, with some reservations, that people could in principle fend off the usual diseases of old age and considerably extend their life span by following a special diet."

It was true. Science believed that if CR could work for monkeys, with whom we share 93 percent genome alignment (compared to only 40 percent with mice), then it should also work for us. Unfortunately, this excitement was somewhat short-lived in the culmination of the second trial from the group of scientists at NIA. In the article published in *Nature*, this team of scientists, led by Julie A. Mattison, Donald K. Ingram, and Rafael de Cabo, reported that they had found no appreciable difference in life span when comparing the calorically restricted and the ad libitum–fed monkeys (meaning they were fed as often as they desired). All hope was not lost, however. An interesting trend emerged from the data to suggest that although life span did not seem affected, healthspan was improved. In fact, among older monkeys, CR seemed to improve components of metabolic health, like triglyceride levels, glucose, and cholesterol, similar to what had been observed in the Bio-spherians. The calorically restricted monkeys also seemed to remain disease-free for longer, with an increase in median healthspan of about 2.5 years.

While the CR impact on life span in monkeys did not agree between the two studies, an interesting observation emerged from the data. The two calorie-restricted groups actually had similar life spans (28.5 years for NIA and 28.3 years at UW). Yet the big differences seemed to stem from the controls, who at NIA reached a median life span of 29.1 years and at UW only attained a median life span of 25.9 years.

In order to untangle the source of the contrasting results, the group of scientists from NIA joined forces with members of the group at UW (led by Dr. Rozalyn Anderson) to write a commentary that meticulously detailed the similarities and differences between the two studies when it came to the survival results, changes in body weight, the food intake and composition, and the resulting physiological and pathological changes exhibited by the groups of monkeys at the two facilities. Based on this report, it seemed that the discrepancy in the results could be boiled down to a few key differences in study design. First, in the study at NIA (that found no difference in life span), the control monkeys, who exhibited a fairly long median life span, were not actually fed ad libitum, but rather they were fed a specified amount that was estimated based on age and size. The calorie-restricted monkeys at NIA were then fed 70 percent of this amount (based on age, sex, and body size). At UW, the control monkeys were essentially free-fed (during the day, but restricted at night). When comparing the reported daily caloric intake of the two groups, it did appear that the monkeys at NIA were eating less than those at UW (about 14 percent less in fact), and perhaps were under a moderate CR diet or, at the very least, not an excess caloric diet.

The second big distinction reflected the differences in the character-istics of the monkeys at the two locations. For instance, at NIA, CR was studied in two separate groups; one for which CR was started in early life and another for which it was started in late life. Conversely, the intervention at UW commenced when all monkeys were about eight years of age (the approximate age at which rhesus monkeys reach developmental maturity). The monkeys also came from diverse origins. Those used by NIA had been born and raised in several locations around the world, with ancestral roots in both India and China, while the UW study included only monkeys born and raised at the Wisconsin National Primate Research Center, all of whom were of Indian origin. Diversity in monkey origin contributed to a substantial difference in the genetic background between the two studies, and interestingly, prior data from mice already pointed to the possibility that the effects of CR and differential tolerance of deficit severity might be genetically determined. For instance, a study looking at mice from dozens of different strains found that calorie restriction did not seem to have equivalent effects across all groups. Rather, it appears that even with calorie restriction, individual differences may drive the benefits we see from various lifestyles.

The third, and perhaps biggest, distinction between the two studies boiled down to the composition of the food. When the diet of the monkeys was decided back in the 1980s, the UW team settled on a diet consisting of twice as much fat than what was selected at NIA (10 percent by weight, versus 5 percent). The diet at UW also had slightly less protein than the diet at NIA, and the protein sources differed—at UW, protein was derived from lactalbumin (a derivative of milk), while at NIA, protein was sourced from a combination of soybean and fish meal. Although the amount of carbohydrates eaten by monkeys at the two locations were comparable, they were obtained from very different sources. At NIA, carbohydrates came from wheat, corn, and only a small percentage from sucrose (6.8 percent), also known as table sugar. By contrast, almost half of the carbohydrates provided to monkeys at UW were from sucrose (45 percent) while the remaining was from corn and dextrin. What this suggests is that the diet at UW was comparable to what we now commonly think of as a Western diet, with high amounts of sugar, refined vegetable oils (with a 46:1 omega-6 to omega-3 ratio), and proteins derived predominantly from animal sources. While not perfect, the diet of controls and calorie-restricted monkeys at NIA was more akin to a pescatarian diet, with low table sugar but high starch content, and both proteins and fats derived from fish and soy.

The differences in the dietary composition between the two monkey trials may explain why one "worked" and one didn't. For instance, there was a big difference when it came to the amount of things like sucrose in each of the diets. Sucrose (table sugar) is a disaccharide, meaning that it consists of one glucose molecule and one fructose molecule. After digesting sucrose, the body breaks it down and the glucose and fructose are then metabolized slightly differently. Glucose will enter the bloodstream very quickly and stimulate the rapid release of insulin so that cells can absorb it immediately. This is not necessarily a bad thing; glucose is the main energy source for our bodies, and our cells use it constantly in order to function. When the available amounts exceed necessary levels (possibly as was the case for control animals at UW), though, glucose will be converted to glycogen and stored in the liver and muscles for short-term use, or converted to fatty acids and stored in adipose tissue (what we think of as our fat cells). Excess amounts of fatty acids from glucose can also be directed to the liver, potentially contributing to a condition called "nonalcoholic fatty liver disease" (NAFLD). Conversely, while fructose contains the same number of calories per gram as glucose or sucrose, it does not elicit a rapid spike in blood sugar and insulin excretion after being ingested.

So what does this mean for us? While the monkey studies provided the tiniest glimmer of hope when it came to the promise of CR in humans, it did not amount to the overwhelming reassurance we were looking for. In many ways, we aren't any closer to determining whether a lifetime of moderate hunger is worth it in the end. That clearly has not stopped some CR enthusiasts from taking a chance on it, though.

THE HUMAN CR EXPERIENCE

Michael Rae is a science writer for the SENS Research Foundation—an organization headed by famed biogenerontologist Dr. Aubrey de Grey and CEO James O'Neill. The foundation focuses on funding opportunities and active research into the biology of aging, with an emphasis on discovering regenerative strategies to counter the threat of age-related diseases. Michael doesn't just write about the potential malleability in the rate of aging through his work with SENS, he is attempting to demonstrate it within himself. While in his early twenties, Michael recalls coming to the realization that our rate of biological aging is not something autonomous or beyond our control. As he bore witness to the decline and death of the people he loved, like his grandparents, he came to view biological aging as "a completely unacceptable horror that was already imperceptibly underway in [his] body and those of everyone around [him], which if left to run its course, would inevitably culminate in disability, disease, dementia, and death." Rather than feeling helpless as he contemplated his own mortality, he used this dread to spur his mission to take back some control. His quest was not immortality, but rather the potential to achieve maybe a decade or so more of healthy life.

Back in the mid-1990s it still wasn't believed that humans could actually sustain a CR diet. So, like most people during that time, Michael was focused on practicing some of the science-backed approaches of the day—eating a low-fat diet with nutritional supplements, exercising, and antioxidant megadosing. At the time, it was believed that available supplements could simulate the benefit of CR, meaning that they could mimic the effects of CR without the hunger requirement. As an already slender individual, Michael initially saw this as an ideal solution. With time, though, it became apparent that nothing being developed showed any appreciable benefits or were scientifically credible solutions for slowing aging, aside from one—CR.

After what Michael describes as nearly a decade of wasted time and money, he transitioned from the fad diet of the time (high-carb, low-fat, low-protein) to the Zone diet (which requires a daily intake of 40 percent calories from carbs, 30 percent from fat, and 30 percent from protein), and eventually to a Zone-like CR routine. Michael soon found the CR Society, where he quickly became an active member and eventually a member of their board. Through their LISTSERV, he was able to meet like-minded CR subscribers and share tips, science, and general support. In the early 2000s, he witnessed a surge in public enthusiasm for the practice as interest in aging research began to take off in general and the stories of various members of the CR Society were profiled by the media. This peaked as the first nonhuman primate study results from UW were published. Michael reports that enthusiasm has been on the decline ever since, though, starting with the publication of the negative results in the NIA monkey trial and additional overshadowing by study results of pharmaceuticals like rapamycin, or dietary practices like fasting.

Now, as Michael turns fifty, the question remains whether his decades of restricted eating have paid off. Of course, there is no way of comparing the counterfactual—determining what would have happened to Michael's body had he indulged in a standard Western diet, or even a relatively healthy version of one for that matter—but he does appear to be doing better than most others his age. While on the border of being designated as "underweight" by traditional standards, Michael seems to be the picture of health when it comes to his lab tests. He appears to have exceptional cardiovascular health as indicated by his low blood pressure and carotid-femoral pulse wave velocity (which evaluates how stiff a person's arteries are). Arterial stiffening is another phenomenon that occurs with aging and is known to increase a person's immediate risk of conditions such as heart disease, stroke, and even dementia. Additionally, when Michael entered his lab results into the clinical biological age calculator based on the measure I had developed in 2018, the biological age he received was more than a decade younger than what was listed on his driver's license. And he's not alone. Studies of individuals undergoing long-term, self-imposed CR suggest that these individuals exhibit signs of slower aging, similar to what has been observed in many of the animal studies. Overall, they seem to look better on multiple factors associated with risk of cardiovascular disease and/or cancer. They exhibit better lipid profiles and reduced signs of oxidative stress, and they are able to avoid systemic inflammation and maintain insulin sensitivity. Taken together, these adaptations seem to reflect a reduction in the onset of age-related pathology, which should translate to more disease-free years of life in the future.

But as I mentioned before, the problem with studying the benefits of CR in a group of individuals who have self-selected to practice this somewhat extreme regimen for decades is that people like Michael are not average. It takes an enormous amount of discipline coupled with perseverance to overcome our inclination to fill up on food. Evolution has primed our brains to continually seek nutrition. Our ancestors procured food by hunting and gathering, and for that reason it was often in short supply. On the lucky occasion that the tribe was able to track and kill a large prey animal, indulgence (and what we might call gluttony today) was necessary. No one knew when the next big meal would come along. For this reason, our brains became conditioned to seek out calorically dense and/or sweet foods. When we are eating salty, fatty, or sugary things, the neurotransmitter system in our brains reinforces this behavior by inducing a sense of euphoria, which we then associate with the act of eating those kinds of treats.

Yet in people like Michael, the determination to starve off aging pushes them to overcome these urges to eat, even when confronted with hunger pangs. Beyond the pleading from their brains, self-imposed calorie restrictors also have to persevere in the presence of societal pressure. Michael describes the difficulty in maintaining his lifestyle choice in the face of disapproval from friends and family. Eating is as much a social endeavor as it is a physiological one. Michael believes that humans have adapted a propensity not only to want to be together during meals, but also a need to share the bounty. The fact that the typical Western diet (both in terms of nutritional content and proportion) does not facilitate the practice of CR has made social events difficult for many CR enthusiasts. Michael describes how he is often confronted with dissatisfaction when he makes the decision to join a meal with others for the conversation, but not the food. Similarly, when hosts invite you over to their home for dinner, they may view your request to supply your own meal as insulting.

This is all to say that the motivation needed to sustain a CR lifestyle probably also translates to other facets of practitioners' lives. Therefore, one problem with attributing health success to CR alone is that people who engage in the practice are driven to be as healthy as possible, so this may extend to most of the lifestyle choices they make. For instance, Michael is someone who also religiously tracks his sleep and activity. He also actively thinks about aging a lot, as someone who works in the field, and has been trying to intervene in the process for most of his life. While each of us could do what Michael has done—adopt a CR lifestyle and track how this may be impacting our aging profiles—most people need more convincing to even consider the switch. They want to know that it will pay off: that it will work for someone like them; and the only way to estimate that is a clinical trial in humans.

THE HUMAN TRIAL

Enter CALERIE. During the time that scientists were debating the conflicting results from decades-long monkey trials, a new study was moving headlong into the space. This was not just another scientific study of the effects of diet on longevity in another animal model. It was a randomized control trial of CR in humans! The Comprehensive Assessment of Long-Term Effects of Reducing Intake of Energy (CALERIE) started as a collaborative effort among scientists at Tufts University in Boston, Washington University in St. Louis, and Louisiana State University in Baton Rouge. At the onset, the goal of the trial was simply to determine whether people could adhere to a CR diet. Unlike a drug trial, the researchers were dependent on study participants not just volunteering, but actually following through. Subjects would need the willpower to maintain CR for the duration of the two-year trial. To test whether this would be possible, the team enrolled just under fifty volunteers and randomly assigned them to one of four intervention groups. This initial trial was only designed to last twelve months and was meant to determine feasibility of the larger trial.

The control group was put on a diet based on the American Heart Association's Step 1 dietary composition that was meant to match their estimated calorie expenditure. The idea was that controls would not overeat or undereat, but instead ingest the calories needed to maintain their current weight. The second group was a 25 percent CR group. These individuals received the same general makeup of nutrients as the controls, but with only three-quarters of the total calories per day. The third group was a CR group (12.5 percent reduced calories) who were also asked to exercise, such that their total caloric deficit for the day would reach 25 percent of the controls. The idea was that they would only moderately reduce food intake but simultaneously boost caloric needs via physical activity. For instance, for someone requiring 2,000 kcal/day to maintain their weight, this would mean consuming 1,750 kcal/day and engaging in 250 calories worth of additional exercise (something equivalent to a 2.5-mile run every day). The final group was put on an extreme low-calorie liquid diet (890 kcal/day) consisting of four nutrition shakes and one brownie each day. This diet was followed only until subjects had lost 15 percent body weight, after which they were switched to a weight-maintenance diet.

The food for each of the diets was provided for the first three months, after which, participants were asked to adhere to their diets but were permitted to eat foods they bought and prepared themselves. Everyone in the study was required to document what they had eaten on a daily basis. If they ate an extra apple or drank an extra glass of wine (participants in all but the low-calorie liquid diet were permitted some alcohol), they had to report it, along with any perceived reason for deviating from their prescribed plan.

When the data were finally in, it seemed that, perhaps surprisingly, people could be counted on to maintain a CR diet, at least for the short term. The researchers report very few deviations or loss of adherence. Even when individuals did report straying from their prescribed diet, the calorie differential was minor. You might be thinking, "What if they lied? How many people would admit to eating a pint of ice cream when they knew scientists were counting on them?" The beautiful thing about a CR study is that it is actually fairly easy to determine how much someone is in fact eating. It all comes back to the impact of calories in, calories out on weight loss. According to results, the control group only experienced a 0.2 percent decrease in weight over the six-month intervention. This would be equivalent to about 4 pounds in someone weighing 200 pounds at the onset of the study. Conversely, those in the two CR groups (with and without exercise) lost just under 10 percent body weight (or 20 pounds for someone starting at 200 pounds). Finally, for the low-calorie liquid diet group, the average weight loss was just over 13 percent (more than 25 pounds for someone starting at 200 pounds).

With the promising Phase 1 feasibility results under their belt, the research team began their in-depth trial of CR in humans. They enrolled nearly 250 healthy volunteer men and women between the ages of twenty-one and fifty. An important factor was that all participants were not obese at baseline, given that the team wanted to ensure that positive results were not simply attributable to reductions in obesity prevalence. Unlike the Phase 1 trial, Phase 2 only had two groups—a control group that was told to simply maintain their current dietary practice, and a CR group that was allowed to eat what they pleased as long as they reduced their caloric intake by 25 percent. At the end of the study, it was found that, on average, the CR group was only able to achieve a 12 percent reduction in calories over the two-year trial. Even this minor deficit, however, appeared to show promising outcomes. Overall, subjects on the CR diet maintained weights that were 10 percent lower than baseline over the entire two years of the trial. They also generally exhibited reductions in inflammatory markers and improvements in many cardiovascular risk factors. But one of the most exciting findings was their reduction in biological aging.

Using a biological age measure I had developed in 2013, Dr. Daniel Belsky, a colleague at Columbia University, showed that people in the control group (who maintained their normal diets) increased in biological age as expected, or slightly slower than expected. For instance, over the two-year period, they gained about a year and a half of biological age. This might suggest that they were aging slightly slower than what is seen on average in the general population. That still didn't come close to what was observed in the CR group, though. According to results, those assigned to a CR diet only gained about three months of biological age over the entire two-year period. They were aging 87.5 percent slower than we would expect for the average person.

To demonstrate the potential implications of this, let's imagine one of the CALERIE participants. We can call her Isabel. When Isabel enrolls in CALERIE, she is thirty years old chronologically and, according to her lab values, also thirty years old biologically. Isabel ends up getting assigned to the CR arm of the intervention trial. As someone who was lightly active prior to the trial, Isabel was able to maintain her

150-pound frame on about 2,000 kcal/day. During the trial, she is able to successfully reduce her caloric intake to 1,700 kcal/day, which results in a 20-pound weight loss over the two years. More important, at the end of the trial, Isabel's biological age has only increased to 30.5 years, despite the fact that she is now thirty-two years old. This improvement sparks Isabel to adopt a long-term CR lifestyle in which she maintains a daily diet of about 1,800 kcal/day. Four decades later, Isabel decides to retest her biological age to determine the benefits of her adherence to CR. Even if Isabel's biological aging rate picked up again such that she was gaining six months of biological age for every year of chronological age (compared to what was half of that during CALERIE), on her seventieth birthday, Isabel would be gifted with the news that she was only 49.5 years old biologically. Of course, there may be a floor effect. We don't know if it is possible for a seventy-year-old to truly have a biological profile of someone more than twenty years their junior. But the important thing is that slowing the rate of aging will have compounding effects over time.

THE OTHER SIDE OF THE COIN

But what about older individuals? Is there a point when it is too late to start an intervention like CR? While CALERIE only included participants under the age of fifty, studies from rodents and other model animals suggest that CR can extend longevity even when started later in life. There is an important caveat, however, that seems to be emerging from the data—the benefits seem to only occur in individuals who are able to maintain some degree of body weight. Wasting away in response to CR (particularly in older individuals) might actually signify a detrimental response to CR, representing malnourishment or an inability to absorb the nutrients necessary to maintain functioning. As with many things, there seems to be a sweet spot, or Goldilocks effect, in which low calories is good but too low is problematic.

In addition to malnourishment, there are other maladaptive changes that can occur in animals or people who are chronically calorically restricted. Even if malnutrition is not present, significant reductions in caloric intake seem to drive down metabolic rates and reduce levels of something called "leptin." This is notable because leptin is the hormone in your body that signals satiety and in turn reduces feelings of hunger. While for people like Michael Rae, feelings of hunger are a worthy sacrifice for the potential benefits CR might bestow, there are clearly others for whom that is not the case. In addition to feeling hungry, some individuals on CR diets also self-report lower libido, which is likely explained by the observed reductions in circulating sex hormones. Specifically, males on a CR diet have been shown to have substantially lower testosterone levels. There is also evidence that CR may impair immune responses, like wound healing, and cause an individual to be more susceptible to threats of pathogen infection. As mentioned before, it is believed that CR works by essentially turning off (or at least turning down) certain processes. One of these may be the body's immune response. While, overall, the decrease in immune activation may be beneficial for health, given that it will likely result in decreasing systemic inflammation or preventing an overactive immune response in the face of chronic everyday stressors, when problems do arise that call for a robust immune system, you may be out of luck.

Finally, despite the promising success of CR, perhaps one of the biggest problems is that it is really hard to convince a large majority of people to eat 10 to 25 percent less. In most countries, it is hard enough to prevent overeating, let alone promote undereating. While there may be a few among us, like Michael and other CR Society members, who can successfully sustain a CR diet long-term, many of you reading this might not see this as a viable option when it comes to your lifestyle. That doesn't mean it needs to be all or nothing, though. There are other options with appreciable benefits when it comes to slowing aging and preventing major diseases. In fact, the cutting-edge research coming out is starting to suggest that many of them might come close, or even mimic, the benefits seen in CR.

7

Longevity Diets

With so much focus on the impact of diet on aging, does it all just come back to weight, or more specifically body fat? There is no denying that practices like CR will contribute to drastic weight loss, and most people who engage in the habit do maintain a very low body mass index, or BMI. Still, the idea that the only thing that matters for health and aging in the adage of "calories in, calories out" is inherently flawed. What's more, the way we approach the topic of body composition and health has major issues, many of which prevent us from actually helping people achieve healthier, happier lives.

BMI is the ratio of how much we weigh (in kilos) versus how tall we are (in meters squared). In the United States, the average woman is five feet four inches (or 1.63 meters) and weighs 170 pounds (or 77.1 kilos), putting her at a BMI just shy of 30. By today's standards, she is overweight and borderline obese—we classify a BMI over 25 as overweight and a BMI over 30 as obese. But is it really true that everyone with these body stats is on the precipice of obesity? Probably not. These cutoffs that we give so much weight to (excuse the pun) are based on population averages, not on individual specifications. In fact, some bodies are healthier at a BMI of

29, while others are healthier at a BMI of 19. As with most things, it depends on the individual, their genetics, and their unique body composition. So if you are one of those people who has always struggled to maintain a BMI below 25, maybe you don't have to. But how do you know if that is the case? I want to be careful and not suggest that we shouldn't study obesity in the context of health. A large majority of people worldwide are at increased risk of adverse disease and functioning outcomes due to their weight. Instead of focusing so much on a person's pants size or the number on the scale, however, we should be turning our attention to quantitative measures of health and disease risk. Recently, my research has found that when we account for differences in biological age, the link between BMI and health outcomes (like disease risk or mortality) disappears. In some cases, it reverses, suggesting that for two people with the exact same biological age and chronological age, the one with the higher BMI might have a slight (albeit insignificant) health advantage. This is because the way in which things like obesity impact health is by accelerating the aging process. So instead of using someone's weight to serve as a reflection of their health, why don't we just measure it directly?

Imagine that instead of a New Year's resolution to lose ten pounds, we have a resolution to slow our biological aging by a given amount. If we do the things needed for that, like eating nutritiously and not overconsuming calories, our body will likely find the weight that is right for it. We may not all end up looking like the model society has deemed "ideal," but that is probably good because in the end, we will be better off in terms of health and wellness. This way of approaching weight and health is indeed a paradigm shift. Traditionally, and still today, diets have been geared toward helping people lose weight—often as quickly as possible. Popular diets like Paleo, low-carb, or Atkins, which famously hit the diet scene in the 1970s, promised to help people drop lots of pounds fast. For instance, Dr. Robert Atkins claimed subscribers to his diet could lose fifteen pounds in the first two weeks. Whether that is true or not, the enduring popularity of low-carb diets stemmed from their often dramatic weight loss results. Not to mention, dieters were still permitted to consume some of their favorite indulgent foods, like cheese, bacon, and hamburgers (sans bun).

The resulting trends associated with these types of diets were not all good news, however. Recent research is finding that slashing carbohydrate intake may actually shorten your life span. After all, those carbs are replaced with something, and for most people, that something is protein, especially animal protein. New data have linked the consumption of high amounts of animal protein to aging and disease. Despite the myth that carbohydrates are the main culprit when it comes to things like diabetes, heart disease, and cancer, my lab and others have shown that in fact it is the consumption of animal products (like meat and dairy) that may be most dangerous to your health. The reason many people don't realize this is because, in our society, low weight or body mass is often conflated with health.

As a biomedical researcher who has published peer-reviewed papers on obesity, I can't say that the "obesity epidemic" that has occurred in much of the world is not a public health threat. But at the same time, it is not one-to-one. The relationship between weight and health, or aging for that matter, is a more complicated story and, in many instances, having a higher BMI does not always equal worse health, especially when we start thinking about long-term effects on life span and healthspan. To understand this better, one must first unpack the links between body fat and health, while also critically considering what a measure of body mass index truly represents.

FAT CELL SIZE NOT NUMBER

According to a recent study published in *Nature* from Dr. Kirsty Spalding's group at the Karolinska Institutet in Sweden, evidence is starting to show that for adults, the number of fat cells in our bodies (called "adipocytes") may not fluctuate as much as was once believed. This interesting observation instead suggests that as adults, each of us has essentially a set number of fat cells that is unique to us. Some people have more and some people less, but in general your number doesn't change much over the years. Instead, the weight changes that we observe year to year (or month to month) are due more to alterations in the *size* of those cells, rather than the *quantity*.

The study also showed that the number of fat cells each of us has as adults was mostly determined during our early and adolescent development. That is to say, we accumulated fat cells up until around age twenty, at which point, that number became more or less set for each of us. Therefore, the difference between you and me in terms of how many fat cells each of us has today actually resulted from differences acquired growing up, not differences in our current behaviors or lifestyles. In truth, it is likely that many of those differences are due to genetics. This makes sense in light of other so-called anthropometric traits, like height, which are known to be highly genetically determined. It's estimated that 80 percent of the difference between people's heights is explained by differences in genes. While genetic studies of fat cell numbers are more difficult to conduct, similar statics might explain differences between people. Additionally, other factors like biological sex also play a role. On average, women have a higher proportion of body fat than men, which is likely due more to differences in the number of fat cells than the size of each cell.

While the number of fat cells is a major contributor to our overall fat mass and body size, the other part of the equation is the volume—how large and engorged each of our fat cells is. It is this factor that contributes to the fluctuations in weight that a person may experience over time. For instance, if you put on a bit of weight over the winter, you probably didn't do that by accumulating more fat cells, but rather, the ones you already had actually became bigger, denser, and heavier. That being said, while there is some evidence that a very massive and rapid weight gain (or weight gain immediately following weight loss) can cause the body to adjust by increasing the overall number of fat cells—setting a new normal for that individual—most weight gain is due to changes in volume rather than number. Conversely, if you lose weight, this is almost never due to a decrease in the number of fat cells and instead is almost entirely reflective of declines in cell volume. To highlight this, Dr. Spalding's group showed that following bariatric surgery, individuals exhibited a significant decrease in fat cell volume, but showed essentially no changes in the number of fat cells, despite having lost around 18 percent body weight on average. Even in the case of something like liposuction or cryolipolysis, the reduction in fat cells is often short-lived, as the body has developed built-in mechanisms to replenish the cells that were lost. You can't trick your body for the interim—it remembers.

The important thing is to better understand how these two variables (fat cell volume and fat cell number) impact health and aging. For the most part, the majority of adverse outcomes associated with obesity seem to be caused by increases in adipocyte volume and dysfunction, and in many ways, an increased adipocyte number may be benign or even protective. That is because when we eat in excess of our body's needs, those additional nutrients are often stored as lipids (fats) in our adipocytes. As adipocytes become engorged or too full, this will typically trigger a number of maladaptive changes by upregulating things like inflammation and the production of reactive oxygen species or free radicals. Additionally, once adipocyte stores are filled, lipids end up remaining in our circulating blood (often signified by high cholesterol or triglyceride levels). These lipids can go on to damage or alter proteins and other molecular factors. Excess lipids can also be redirected to the liver or pancreas, exacerbating conditions like type 2 diabetes and nonalcoholic fatty liver disease. Given that these phenomena often co-occur, scientists and doctors have developed a term for the simultaneous presence of more than one of these compounding health risks, called "metabolic syndrome." Not surprisingly, metabolic syndrome is associated with a substantial increase in the risk of heart disease, diabetes, and stroke, but additionally it also has been shown to increase risks for many common cancers, as well as for Alzheimer's disease and fatty liver disease.

While on the one hand having "fatter fat cells" is typically problematic, having a greater number of fat cells, on the other hand, isn't innately bad. In fact, humans have the highest proportion of fat cells of all primates, leading some researchers to reference humans as "the fat primate." Most monkeys have below 9 percent body fat, which is similar to what Arnold Schwarzenegger had in 1974 when he became Mr. Olympia. Yet our relative abundance of fat cells, compared to closely related hominids, may be what enabled us to evolve some of our most prized traits. Our large brains and corresponding intellect require tremendous energy supplies to power it. This results in much higher metabolic rates. When our ancestors were able to hunt and kill large animals for meat, their expanded fat cell pools enabled them to store essential energy resources that could be used later or during times when food again became scarce. Our bodies adapted to having high-capacity rechargeable batteries. We don't just use energy sources as they become available; we have optimized the storage of energy far better than our close relatives.

Unfortunately, in modern society, this amazing system hardly ever comes into play. Many people don't encounter long periods of time without food and instead we are at risk of overloading the system, causing engorgement of our fat cells that remain that way and are never depleted. The cycle of fasting and feeding that we evolved to survive is no longer necessary for most people; instead, we engage in continuous feeding. Ironically, this is one reason why having more fat cells may actually be moderately protective, and perhaps is one of many explanations as to why women are on average at lower risk of conditions like diabetes and heart disease. More cells equates to more storage capacity, which means your body has a bigger buffer against excessive consumption. For instance, imagine you have a gallon of water that you need to keep stored in separate cups (maybe you don't have a pitcher). If you have only ten cups, each one will be quite full. However, if you have twenty cups, the water can be distributed and each individual cup will be less full.

Fat can also be distributed across cells in different ways. This is important because where the excess fat accumulates seems to have a major impact on health. Accumulation of lipids within (1) visceral fat, which is the fat surrounding organs, or (2) ectopic fat, which refers to fat stored in cells that are not adipocytes (usually in the liver, muscles, or pancreas), contributes to greater metabolic disorder, systemic inflammation, and overall physiological dysregulation than does fat stored in subcutaneous regions, which is the fat just under the skin. Thus, having more subcutaneous fat, as is the case for women compared to men, on average, might mean that less fat has to be diverted to problematic regions.

Unfortunately, having more fat cells can be an issue if individuals engage in overconsumption. It can also make people more likely to regain weight directly following a major weight reduction. While having engorged or high-volume fat cells causes metabolic and inflammatory problems, depleted fat cells can elicit hormonal changes that drive feelings of hunger. This of course makes sense given that hunger is your body's way of telling you that you need to replenish or recharge the empty backup batteries. This is one explanation as to why obese individuals who lose a lot of weight fairly quickly often struggle to keep it off. Again, losing weight will not decrease the number of fat cells; it will just empty them. As the storage of fat in adipocytes is diminished, these cells stop secreting the hormone leptin. Production of less leptin triggers the part of the brain called the "hypothalamus" that it's time to eat! Leptin can be thought of as a sensor and/or regulator of your energy intake and storage. It is the way fat cells signal to the brain that energy stores are running low and you need to find food to replenish them (when leptin is turned off). Conversely, it also tells your body when enough resources are stored, signaling that you can stop searching for food, at least until they become depleted again. The amount each of us needs to eat to get to that level will vary due to a few things, one being our metabolic rate, or essentially how fast we use up the food/energy being consumed, and another being the number of fat cells the energy stores are distributed across, which will determine how full each individual cell gets. The more cells we have, the less full each is, and the more food our body signals that it needs.

Because of this, individuals with more fat cells may actually have a much harder time maintaining a low BMI. As an example, imagine two people of the same height and the same weight, yet one has 20 percent more fat cells than the other. In order for them to weigh the same amount, the person with more fat cells would also have to have much smaller (or more depleted) fat cells. In turn, the person with more, but smaller fat cells would likely produce less leptin, and thus feel hungrier. As you can imagine, it might be harder for them to maintain their current weight in the face of constant opposition from their brain. We have to ask ourselves again, however, whether these two people should weigh the same. In reality, the one with more fat cells might do better at a slightly higher weight. Again, I am not promoting excess obesity, just stating that what we define as a healthy weight should be personalized to our unique characteristics.

Yet rather than trying to determine differences in fat cell numbers to infer something about personalized differences in natural weight propensity, a better tactic is to simply throw weight out the window and instead switch our focus to estimates of health—things like biological age. By switching our focus to optimizing health and aging, and doing all the things that best serve that goal, we should end up at a weight that is right for each of us. Yes, some of us will be heavier, while others lighter, but what is most important is that we are all healthier.

DIETS TO SLOW AGING

When it comes to traditional diets, two have emerged as front-runners for promoting healthy aging. These include the plant-based or vegan diet and the Mediterranean diet. While it is not hard to imagine that a diet rich in leafy green vegetables will be beneficial for health and aging, the focus on a plant-based diet for promoting longevity actually emerged from research focused on CR.

During the early twenty-first century, studies in yeast, worms, and rodents started to demonstrate that a reduction in specific nutrients, rather than calorie intake as a whole, was the main contributor to the life span and healthspan benefits seen in the animals undergoing CR. The macronutrient at the heart of these findings was protein. Now, if you are, like many individuals, aware of dietary guidelines, you might think that high protein is the way to go. After all, diets like Atkins, Paleo, and in some instances keto, promote the health benefits of low-carb/high-protein for improving muscle functioning and preventing obesity and type 2 diabetes. The data coming out of the laboratories looking at aging, however, were finding that high protein intake was associated with faster aging rates, while low protein (or protein restriction) seemed to mimic the effects of CR. Studies started, in fact, to suggest that protein restriction alone fully accounted for the beneficial effects of CR. In flies, it was shown that reduced protein intake, rather than carbs or total calories, promoted longevity and this could be undone when protein was increased in the diet but not when carbohydrates or fat were.

It was postulated that the reason for this came down to the effects of dietary protein and/or calories on a factor called "IGF-1." IGF-1 is a hormone involved in growth during development and in anaerobic activities throughout life. It is a by-product of a growth hormone, which has been erroneously touted as an antiaging compound. If you google "human growth hormone," you will undoubtedly be faced with images from supplement companies depicting older men with impressive muscular physiques. The truth is that while human growth hormone may facilitate muscle building, it and IGF-1 have been shown time and again to also promote aging and, specifically, cancer. It was thus rationalized that the reduction in IGF-1 in response to CR in rodents or other animals explained the slowing of the aging process and reductions in tumor growth. Yet when scientist Dr. Luigi Fontana from the University of Sydney looked at IGF-1 levels of humans on a CR diet, he observed that they were not decreased unless the composition of the individual's diet was also low in dietary protein. He further showed that humans did not have to restrict calories altogether in order to elicit reductions in IGF-1. All they needed was to eat a plant-based diet that included little to no animal protein.

Adding more evidence to the low protein hypothesis, in 2014, I published a study with Dr. Valter Longo and colleagues suggesting that low protein intake—particularly low animal protein—was associated with a reduction in aging-related risks. In looking at a nationally representative sample of about 3,000 middle-aged Americans, we grouped individuals into three categories based on protein consumption. Those who reported consuming an average of 20 percent or more of their calories from protein sources were designated as the high protein consumption group. Those with less than 10 percent of calories from protein were considered the low protein group, and those who fell somewhere between 10 and 20 percent of calories from protein were designated as having moderate protein consumption. When we compared outcomes for these three groups over nearly twenty years of follow-up, we observed that those in the high protein group had a 74 percent increased risk of dying early than those in the low protein group. When it came to cancer and diabetes, those in the high protein group were far more likely to die of either of these conditions than individuals in the low protein group. The moderate protein group also showed an increased risk (about threefold) when it came to diabetes or cancer mortality as compared to the risks observed in the low protein group.

Again, because this is an observational study in which people are self-selecting to eat a certain way, it is possible that some other extraneous factors could differ between the groups and explain our findings. When we checked for the impact of differences in total caloric intake or other macronutrients, however, none of them explained our results. We also tested whether things like gender, race/ethnicity, education, waist circumference, smoking habits, exercise habits, preexisting conditions, attempts to lose weight, or yo-yo dieting could explain our findings. None of them did. The only two things that seemed to come out of the data were: (1) that the source of protein mattered, and (2) that IGF-1 was likely the culprit. For instance, we showed that most of the effect was explained by high consumption of animal protein, but when we compared that with differences in consumption of plant-based protein, the associated risks went away. High plant-based protein did not seem to be a problem. We also had data on IGF-1 levels measured in the blood of participants. We found that the cancer risk associated with eating a high protein diet was compounded for people with high IGF-1 levels. This meant that the biggest risk was for high protein/high IGF-1, but protein was less detrimental for low IGF-1 individuals.

LET THEM EAT PLANTS

Since our study was published in 2015, a number of other scientific publications have come out touting the benefits of a plant-based or low animal protein diet. In general, most researchers in the field of aging would agree that in general a vegan diet is likely the best option for improving life span and healthspan. Nonetheless, as someone who follows a plant-based diet, I think it is also critical to acknowledge that there are healthy vegan diets and there are certainly unhealthy vegan diets. For instance, some of the most notorious junk foods are in essence vegan. Things like Oreo cookies, certain potato chips, some brownie or cake box mixes, Airheads candies, Hershey's Syrup, and Twizzlers. I doubt anyone would argue that a diet laden with these highly processed, sugary, and salty treats would buy them a longer life. Conversely, a diet composed of whole foods, including vegetables, seeds, nuts, legumes, and whole grains, has the potential to dramatically improve cardiometabolic health, reduce cancer risk, and promote longevity.

Up until very recently, ideas of veganism tended to elicit images of tree huggers and earth mothers, or perhaps card-carrying PETA members, but the plant-based lifestyle has now started to penetrate mainstream culture. A recent report showed that the prevalence of people who identify as being vegan increased 600-fold between 2014 and 2017. Moreover, the influx of meat alternatives have made even the most hardcore burger lovers take a serious look at plant-based living. This was also aided by the reports stating that adoption of a plant-based diet may be one of the most beneficial things an individual can personally do to fight climate change. Yet, despite the growing consensus regarding the benefits of going vegan, for many, this lifestyle still seems unfeasible.

Many people worry that forgoing meat will diminish their stamina and power. Even for those who pursue athletics recreationally, but especially for professionals who depend on their performance for their livelihood, the concern is always whether plants can provide enough fuel and muscle-building nutrients to keep someone at peak performance. Much of this, again, comes back to concerns over protein, given that protein serves as building blocks for our muscles. There is an inherent worry that vegans will need more protein to maintain the same level of performance as their meat-eating counterparts. The truth is, the amount of protein needed will be similar—there are some differences in digestibility of plant versus animal protein, but that should only contribute to a negligible difference in what is absorbed. The more important thing is being strategic in what you eat and where your plant protein sources come from.

Proteins are made up of amino acids, many of which can be generated by our own bodies without the need to digest them. There are nine amino acids, referred to as "essential amino acids," however, that we must get from our diet. Our bodies can't produce them on their own. These are histidine, isoleucine, leucine, lysine, methionine, phenylalanine, threonine, tryptophan, and valine. The protein sources we eat can therefore be designated as either complete proteins, meaning they contain all nine essential amino acids (what most animal proteins are), or incomplete proteins, meaning they lack at least one of the nine essential amino acids. It is important to remember that "essential" doesn't mean these are more important amino acids and so should be consumed in high quantities. Interestingly, methionine and tryptophan (two essential amino acids) have been identified as potentially pro-aging when eaten in high amounts, and some studies have hinted that the benefits seen when animals are placed on either protein restriction or caloric restriction diets are due to the reduced intake of both or one of these essential amino acids. Note that considerably more work needs to be done before people start thinking of barring methionine or tryptophan from their dinner plates completely.

That being said, it is important for athletes and health-conscious people alike to be aware of the protein and other macromolecular content of their meals, in order to ensure they are ingesting a well-balanced and sustainable diet. Contrary to what most people assume, it isn't that hard to devise a plant-based diet that contains all the nutrients necessary to physically succeed in sports. In fact, a number of athletes who have made the switch to plant-based eating have said their performance has never been better. The table on the next page illustrates how anyone can derive suitable protein content simply from plants. On the left are plant-based options that contain complete proteins—all essential amino acids. On the right are plant-based protein sources that for the most part are missing only one or two essential amino acids.

Complete Proteins		Incomplete Proteins	
Quinoa	8 g/cup	Almonds	6 g/oz.
Buckwheat	6 g/cup	Sweet Potatoes	2 g/cup
Edamame	17 g/cup	Black Beans	16 g/cup
Hemp	9 g/oz.	Brown Rice	5 g/cup
Spirulina	64 g/cup	Chickpeas	39 g/cup
Chia Seeds	4.7 g/oz.	Brussels Sprouts	3 g/cup

The important thing to remember is that when we prepare a meal, it usually encompasses a combination of different food sources. So even when the individual foods are not complete protein sources, in many cases your meal still can be. For instance, combining brown rice and beans produces a complete protein meal using two incomplete sources. Another example is Ezekiel bread, which contains four to five grams of plant-based protein per slice. While the individual grains that make up Ezekiel bread are incomplete sources of protein on their own, when combined, each slice contains all nine essential amino acids. Given the versatility in plant-based foods, there is no reason to think that forgoing meat and dairy would jeopardize your PR time or make you less of a threat on the court, field, or in the ring. Just ask famous vegan athletes like Alex Morgan, DeAndre Jordan, Rich Roll, James Wilks, Patrik Baboumian, or Derrick Morgan (among many others).

In addition to concerns about protein, stamina, and strength, the other point of contention people have when it comes to going completely green is that they simply love meat. A lot of people can't imagine a life devoid of some of their favorite savory foods. Also, for many people, preparing and eating certain kinds of food is an important part of their heritage and tradition that they want to keep alive. In the end it is not my place, nor anyone else's, to tell you that you can't or shouldn't eat meat. It comes down to deciding what lifestyle you are willing to embrace in light of knowing the potential health impact of your decisions. Even beyond that—while society places a lot of importance on health, for many people that isn't their number one priority in life. Or at least there is a limit to what each of us is willing to do to optimize our overall health. Therefore, the answer of whether someone should go vegan may come down to how much it is personally worth to them. Would they do it if it would buy them half a year of healthier life? What about ten years? While there is no way to know exactly what these outcomes would be for two distinct lifestyle choices, measuring biological age can shed some light on how much our different life decisions matter.

For many people, it may be enough to eat plant-based, let's say, 75 percent of the time, and they might find that the benefits of doing so are significant without the need to give up something that they may consider an important part of their life. People need tools that will enable them to make a more informed decision, however. Truthfully, when it comes down to it, there isn't only one route to a longer healthspan and life span. There is a combination of different choices we can make, each contributing in different ways to our overall health and aging.

So, can you have your meat and live long too? When we look around the world, the answer seems to be yes (to some extent). It all comes back to the adage of eating in moderation.

THE WISDOM OF THE "BLUE ZONES"

In 2004, *National Geographic* explorer Dan Buettner traveled the world with a group of aging and longevity scientists to study the secrets of remote longevity hot spots around the world. These places, called "Blue Zones," have some of the longest-lived populations in the world, whose members also enjoy lives mostly free from cancer, heart disease, and diabetes. The five Blue Zones—Ikaria, Greece; Okinawa, Japan; Sardinia, Italy; Loma Linda, California; and Nicoya Peninsula, Costa Rica—share a few very important things in common. Perhaps most notable is that the people in these communities consume mostly plant-and-bean-rich diets, low in both meat and dairy . . . although not completely exclusionary. While geographical evidence is not enough to infer causality, it has been shown that when people move away from these communities, they tend to also lose their longevity advantage—suggesting that it is not a difference in genetics, but instead likely has to do with the lifestyle practices in these amazing places.

While there are a number of differences between these unique communities and the ones that many of us live in, scientists and organizations have begun to systematically study the residents living in the Blue Zones with the hope of determining their secrets to longevity. Resulting from the original exploration, the Blue Zones Project was launched in 2009 with the goal of using insights from their studies on Blue Zone residents to help transform communities around the world. One of the most striking of these observations to date has to do with the similarities in dietary patterns across the various Blue Zones. Using nutritional surveys, the researchers showed that individuals in Blue Zones tended to follow a few simple practices.

Even though people living in four out of the five Blue Zones reported that they ate meat, it was generally only in extremely small quantities or on rare occasions. In fact, the data suggested that only about 5 percent of their average daily intake was from animal products, while *most of their diet was derived from plants* (95 percent of calories). This meant they were also not on low-carb diets; instead, about 65 percent of their intake was from carbohydrates, 20 percent from fat, and 15 percent from protein (nearly all plant-based). Three of the Blue Zones consume moderate amounts of dairy. Seventh-Day Adventists living in Loma Linda, California, maintain a vegetarian diet and therefore do not necessarily restrict consumption of animal products other than meat. Like many Americans, they still enjoy cheeses, yogurts, and the occasional glass of milk. In Ikaria, Greece, and Sardinia, Italy, goat and/or sheep farming is a prevalent part of life, and as a result, residents regularly consume yogurts, fermented milks, and cheeses. These versions, however, in many ways may not resemble the highly processed, sugar-laden, and factory-farmed dairy products available in a swath of supermarkets across much of the industrialized world.

Also, the sugar consumption in Blue Zones is a fraction of what is typically seen in other locales. On average, Americans ingest about five times the amount of sucrose (table sugar) as Blue Zone inhabitants. The high sugar consumption across much of the world may be unintentional. It's not that people are sitting around eating boxes of cookies, but unfortunately, added sugar has been incorporated into much of our processed foods—from low-fat yogurts to baked beans and even seemingly healthy salads. The Chinese chicken salad from a popular (not to be named) restaurant in the United States packs 44 grams of sugar in one meal! Even if that was the only thing you consumed in a whole day, that would still be twice the added sugar that is eaten daily in Blue Zones. In addition to meals, snacks also distinguish Blue Zone residents from the rest of us. Between meals, people in these areas often turn to plant-based whole foods like fruits and veggies, and especially nuts. In Ikaria, residents reach for a handful of almonds when hungry. In Nicoya, it's pistachios.

Taken together, the diets in Blue Zones look a lot like Mediterranean diets, but with a majority (95 percent) plant-based focus. It is essentially a healthy, unprocessed, whole-food vegetarian or vegan diet, but with some allowance for occasional meat and/or dairy products. As such, this may actually be a diet that is feasible for a lot of people around the world. It offers options, without stringent restrictions, and is not framed in an "all or nothing" context. Followers of the diet are allowed to celebrate with their favorite traditional meals, so long as they limit those to special occasions. This might mean eating vegetarian six days a week (with limited dairy intake) and saving one day a week for meat consumption (ideally, free-range unprocessed meats). It all comes down to moderation. It also means, however, that the majority of foods you are eating are things like vegetables, potatoes, whole grains, nuts, seeds, limited no-sugar-added full-fat dairy products, rice, beans, and olive oil. To quench your thirst, beverages are limited to water, coffee, and tea. The occasional glass of wine seems to be okay too.

Finally, one of the other critical lessons on the diets in these remarkable regions is not so much focused on what you eat, but how you think about food consumption. Buettner describes a Confucian teaching embraced by the people of Okinawa, Japan (the region with the highest female longevity and the highest proportion of centenarians in the world). "*Hara hachi bun me*" roughly translates to "belly 80 percent full" in English. By following this teaching, Okinawans tend to consume only 1,800 to 1,900 calories a day and maintain BMIs in the low 20s throughout their lives. Many researchers have speculated that this moderate, lifelong caloric restriction may actually be what explains the remarkable life expectancies in Okinawa and many of the other Blue Zones.

FASTING FOR LIFE

So are we back at square one? Does this just reaffirm that the path to a long, healthy life is via decades of major reductions in food consumption? Scientists have speculated that while traditional caloric restriction might be the most optimal or straightforward diet for increasing life span and delaying disease, it's perhaps not the only option. Over the past few years, there has been a growing buzz about a dietary regimen that is threatening to replace caloric restriction as the preeminent longevity diet: the practice of fasting. Proponents of various fasting diets claim that it can produce most of the same benefits of a CR diet, but with a very important distinction—it's easier to maintain. In fact, there is good evidence that fasting is in many ways just "CR lite."

Fasting is also a major way of life in Blue Zones. On the 99-square-mile Greek island of Ikaria, residents engage in a number of healthy behaviors that may account for their long lives. They consume locally sourced, organic foods, much from the vegetables grown in their gardens and shared among the community. They partake in continuous physical activity, not in the ways many of us do, but because they live on a hilly island and walking ends up being a major mode of transportation for them. Another interesting observation that Buettner made, though, was that Ikarians fast—a lot. This is because Ikarians follow the Greek Orthodox practices of religious fasting, or "nistia." Every year Ikarians can be observed fasting around 150 days, which include the 40-day Christmas fast; the 48-day Lent fasts; the Fast of Holy Apostles, lasting between 8 and 42 days; and the two-week fast of the Dormition of the Virgin Mary. Additionally, the majority of Wednesdays and Fridays throughout the year are designated fasting days (unless they fall on major feast days). These sacred times are not marked by complete fasts (similar to what is seen during the daylight hours of the Muslim holy month of Ramadan, or the Jewish Day of Atonement, Yom Kippur), but observers instead abstain from certain food groups, mostly meat, dairy, fish, and occasionally oil. While these fasts do not directly restrict calories, researchers have shown that fasters typically incur deficits of about 300 calories a day as compared to those who do not fast during these times. While seemingly small, over a single year, this would equate to about 45,000 fewer calories.

The practice of fasting has a long history dating back to ancient Egyptian, Greek, Chinese, and Indian civilizations. While fasting often aligns with religious and spiritual observances, historical accounts also suggest that it was used as a curative practice to promote health, healing, and renewal. During the sixth century BC, the famous mathematician and philosopher Pythagoras sought to increase his creativity and mental fortitude by fasting for forty days straight. Similar routines were also utilized by Plato, Socrates, and Hippocrates. On the other side of the world, during the pre-Qin dynasty, Daoist masters were promoting the practice of *bigu* (辟谷), in which individuals avoided grain and instead subsisted on very small quantities of raw foods (described in the Daoist text *Biographies of the Immortals* [列仙传]), comprising seeds, nuts, resin, sap, bark, and roots. The hypothesis was that through fasting, individuals would not only improve health and wellness but also increase spiritual awareness. It was a first step toward immortality and achieving divinity. Instead of consuming foods, one could derive nourishment from *qi*, defined as "breath," "vital energy," or "spirit," and in doing so, destroy the *sanshi* (三尸, "three corpses") or malignant evils that reside in each of us and seek to initiate sickness and hasten death. Essentially, agents of aging.

These ancient practices that preceded some notions of the modern-day scientific method and our understanding of Western medicine do have merit. New scientific evidence is emerging to suggest that short, sporadic instances of food deprivation may confer similar longevity and health benefits to CR. As I recently heard one scientist state, "Fasting is the new CR." And it's true. Much of what we have learned about the potential benefits of fasting stem from decades of studies of caloric restriction. Not long ago, scientists looking over the CR literature made an interesting observation. For many animal studies, especially in rodents, calories were restricted by feeding animals only once a day.

This then raised the question of whether the effects being seen were solely due to reduced food intake or, conversely, were a result of prolonged periods of fasting. To follow this up, a research group at the National Institute on Aging tested the next logical thing. They put mice on an alternate-day fasting regimen that was not characterized by an overall reduction in calories. Essentially, the mice ate the same amount as they normally would, but within a shorter time window. What they found was that these mice exhibited improvements in glucose levels and insulin sensitivity (markers associated with diabetes). They also showed that the neuronal cells in the brains of fasted mice were better protected against damage when subjected to toxic stressors. Also, similar to the animals on CR, fasted mice showed reduced risk factors for cardiovascular disease and stroke.

What's more, the benefits are not just observed in rodents. Recently, Dr. Mark Mattson—a scientist at the National Institute on Aging and a pioneer in the CR and intermittent fasting fields—has remarked on how bodybuilders have in many cases stumbled on the benefits of fasting for improving their physiques almost by accident. They have learned through trial and error that skipping breakfast and then working out while fasting helped to decrease body fat while simultaneously building lean mass. The result . . . significant muscle definition and a better chance at success in their sport.

This practice is also backed up by emerging science. A 2013 study showed that when paired with endurance exercise, obese individuals who undertook alternate-day fasting for three months lost substantial fat mass, while retaining muscle mass. What's more, they also saw significant improvements in their cholesterol levels, marked by decreases in LDL (the bad cholesterol) and increases in HDL (the good cholesterol).

In the coming years, more and more clinical trials on fasting are set to come out that will shape our understanding of the potential benefits of this practice. Much of the boom in studies of fasting in humans is because, in contrast to CR, which has been studied for decades in animals with little investigation in humans, the proposed fasting diet is seen by many as being significantly more feasible. People have less trouble incorporating fasting as part of their lifestyle, and it is much easier to recruit study participants—and perhaps more important, retain them.

While scientists have been able to administer a CR diet to animals in the laboratory, there is no way to ensure human participants will comply, even for a study lasting only a few years. While Biosphere 2 showed us humans can subsist on CR, and perhaps even thrive, it is our resilience in the face of our evolutionary drive to eat that ultimately gets in the way. That being said, in fasting studies, subjects often only have to maintain willpower for short bouts of time—a few hours a day or a few days a week.

This also explains why fasting has become so popular in general. It promises the results of CR, without the commitment to a life of sustained hunger. While avid CR practitioners promise that your body will adjust to the deprivation, most people don't have the willpower to ever reach that point. That appears not to be the case with fasting. According to a survey by the International Food Information Council, intermittent fasting was the most popular diet of 2018. Once considered a fad, fasting has quickly become the go-to practice for individuals worried about health and aging. While these diets do also help with weight loss, particularly in overweight or obese individuals, fasting diets also seem to delay or perhaps reverse some of the physical changes of aging.

This past year, I teamed up with two aging researchers and fasting experts, Dr. Valter Longo and Dr. Sebastian Brandhorst, to test the impact of a fasting-mimicking diet (FMD) on biological aging across two clinical trials. While I will describe this and other fasting diets in detail a little later, briefly, FMD is a five-day diet in which individuals do eat, but at very reduced caloric intake (often around 500 calories a day). FMD is typically undertaken once per month or a few times per year. For the first clinical trial, one hundred subjects were randomly assigned to one of two groups. Group 1 was asked to maintain their normal diet for three months, after which they were asked to undertake three cycles of FMD (once per month for three months). Group 2 was asked to start three cycles of FMD from the onset of the study. In the second clinical trial, forty-four subjects with cardiometabolic risk factors at baseline were put on four cycles of FMD over four months. In the second study, there was no control group, but subjects were compared to their baseline states.

As expected, in both clinical trials, those on FMD showed significant reduction in BMI, total fat, subcutaneous fat (the fat under the skin), and visceral fat (the dangerous fat that surrounds vital organs in the abdominal cavity). The most exciting outcome was that it was also shown that FMD reduced hepatic fat fraction, which assesses the proportion of fat in the liver. This is critical given that it reflects risks for nonalcoholic fatty liver disease (NAFLD), which impacts nearly 20 to 30 percent of adults and is linked to early mortality, liver failure, and diabetes. In addition to fat loss, fasting was also associated with improvements in insulin sensitivity and reductions in blood sugar levels. Fasted subjects were found to exhibit more youthful immune profiles following multiple cycles of FMD. But if all these things weren't enough, we also found that FMD subjects were able to reduce their estimated biological age.

Using the measure I had developed (that Dr. Daniel Belsky also applied to the CALERIE data), we showed that after three cycles of FMD, subjects appeared approximately 2.5 years younger than before they started the intervention. That doesn't just suggest that FMD slowed aging, but it actually seemed to reverse it. This was not the case for controls, who after three months of their normal diet showed expected increases in biological age by about half a year. What's more, because we had previously published substantial research to demonstrate the links between a person's biological age and their health risks, we were able to estimate what these reductions meant in terms of possible improvements in long-term health. I want to stress that these are simulated estimates and were not actually observed results (to do that we would have needed a more than fifty-year study). That being said, they are based on sound science and very strong associations. What we found was that between baseline and following the third cycle of FMD, subjects reduced their twenty-year risk of mortality by 30 percent, meaning they were 30 percent less likely to die in the next two decades. Much of this is likely accounted for by the predicted reductions in risks for heart disease (17 percent), cancer (6.5 percent), cerebrovascular disease (22 percent), and diabetes (26 percent). This suggested that FMD doesn't just improve outcomes for specific conditions but, instead, impacts diseases across the board due to its effect on biological aging as a whole.

Despite these exciting results, there are some caveats to consider. The results are, of course, estimates and they assume that the 2.5-year decrease due to three cycles of FMD will be maintained over the long term. That is to say that if a forty-year-old who had a biological age of forty at baseline reduced their biological age to 37.5 years after FMD, when we revisited them again ten years later, they would have a chronological age of fifty, but a biological age of 47.5 years. This is probably not a reality for everyone. Some people will rebound and return to their baseline states if these practices aren't maintained in the long run.

We see this with weight loss programs all the time. For our study, we did check back to see how the subjects' biological ages had changed a few months after the last FMD cycle. Overall, most retained their decrease, but to a lesser extent. That doesn't necessarily tell us what might happen over years or even decades, however. Presumably, the effect of this short intervention would be washed away. But what would happen if people decided to incorporate FMD into their everyday lifestyle? While like before, we didn't have years to figure out the answer, so we turned again to simulations. This time, we simulated what decreases in biological age would look like if someone were to do three cycles every year. Keep in mind, that's only fifteen days of fasting annually, which for most of us is a very achievable endeavor.

To do this, we started with a population of people who were representative of the U.S. population as a whole. This data set, called NHANES, had been collected by the CDC for decades. You can think of it like the U.S. census, but for health. That meant that the people in our sample had similar distributions of demographics, socioeconomic status, geographic diversity, and even comparable biological ages to what one might find if we looked at every adult in the United States. Using our data from the clinical trial, we estimated a predicted change in biological age after three cycles of FMD for everyone ages twenty to fifty in the population. This was based on each person's profile at the onset, while also allowing for some random chance of variation, including the chance that FMD would not decrease biological age in a person (or might even increase it). This also meant that some people were theoretically starting FMD in their twenties, while others were starting in their fifties. Our model also allowed for a moderate "rebound phase" in accordance with our clinical trial data for months when FMD was not practiced.

After finally including all these parameters into the mathematical model, what we found was remarkable. According to our simulation, individuals tended to experience a sharp decrease in biological age after the first year. This meant that, similar to what we observed in the clinical trial, people were getting younger. The next five or so years were followed by almost stagnant biological aging. Year after year, people's biological age appeared frozen in time. Finally, it started to tick up again, but unlike what was expected for a control population, who would be expected to gain one year of biological age for every chronological year that passed, the simulated FMD participants only gained 0.85 years. They were aging at a rate that was 15 percent slower! Overall, these results suggested a possible floor effect when it came to the impact of FMD on biological aging. There is only so much younger you can get and, inevitably, we will all age. We can age more slowly and over time, however, and this will compound into major potential reductions in disease and age-related disability, which in turn may grant us more healthy years of life.

To further test this, we compared everyone who was fifty years old at baseline and simulated two possible scenarios. The first assumed that they would gain one year of biological age for every year they were alive. This is basically what we typically expect. The second scenario used the results from our simulation in which we estimated changes in biological age as a function of undertaking three cycles of FMD annually. Both groups (who were actually the same people, but with two future paths) were simulated for twenty years, at which point we compared their life expectancies and disease risks. The data suggested that twenty years of FMD could buy individuals about five years of life expectancy. What's more, the data suggested that FMD may also help a person achieve better health during that time. The simulated FMD effects suggested that it could reduce heart disease risks by 50 percent, cancer by 30 percent, diabetes by 75 percent, and cerebrovascular disease by 65 percent.

When these results popped up on my computer screen, I found it unbelievable that only one hundred days of partial fasting over a twenty-year period could equate to over 1,800 extra days on this Earth. Not only that, it had the potential to slash a person's risk of developing some of the most loathsome diseases people suffer from as they grow old. Assuming the simulation is accurate, getting people to incorporate intermittent fasting into their lives could have extreme benefits for population health.

Fasting also seems like a much easier "sell" than CR. While the data may not be enough to prompt you to eat 20 percent less indefinitely, many people are encouraged by the idea of simply restricting when they eat, or eating less in short bouts of time. Another advantage of fasting seems to be that it can take on multiple forms, meaning that people have options in determining what works for them. Over the years, there have been more than half a dozen different types of fasting regimens that have been proposed. Currently, there isn't good enough data to suggest which are superior, and it may be the case that some work better for some people than others. The beauty of measures like biological age, however, is that people can try different options. We have shown that these measures can provide fairly quick feedback. This would, therefore, allow people to test which routines work well for their lifestyle and overall health. There is no one-size-fits-all and it really is up to each person (with input from their physician) to determine the right fit.

If you are someone interested in trying out fasting or just curious to hear what it actually entails, here are a few versions that researchers are looking at for their longevity benefits:

Fasting-Mimicking Diet (FMD)

FMD is a regimen discovered and developed by Dr. Valter Longo. It is what was used in the clinical trial where we observed improvement in biological age following three cycles. In FMD, each cycle consists of a five-day, low-calorie diet, in which participants consume about 4,500 kcals over the entire five-day period. The cycle is meant to ease individuals into the restricted calorie regimen, such that, on day 1, individuals will eat just over 1,000 kcal, consisting of 11 percent protein, 46 percent fat, and 43 percent carbohydrates. By day 2, and for the remaining days, however, this is reduced to just over 700 kcal per day with 9 percent of calories coming from protein, 44 percent fat, and 47 percent carbohydrates.

While, hypothetically, one could construct a DIY FMD by preparing your own foods, Dr. Longo stresses that FMD has only been rigorously tested using the pre-specified plant-based food sources, made up mostly of soups, tea, and bars that are supplied as part of the trademarked Pro-Lon diet, available through the company's website. Based on empirical data, it is suggested that people complete three five-day cycles (usually one cycle per month) whenever "you are looking for rejuvenation." While some have complained about the high price tag, given the amount of food provided, the company also offers a reduced price for low-income individuals who qualify. (As a note, I work with Dr. Longo, but have no financial incentives to promote FMD.)

Alternate-Day Fasting (ADF)

Feast or famine. Perhaps, like our ancestors experienced, ADF is characterized by days of food scarcity or complete fasting, followed by free feeding or eating until satiated. As with FMD, the modified version involves minimal consumption, around 500 calories per day, on fasting days, with the alternative days being "unrestricted." While many health professionals worry that this routine could reinforce binge-eating habits on non-fasted days, studies are showing that it can help overweight or obese individuals who want to lose weight. Moreover, similar to the other intermittent fasting protocols, data from lab tests suggest that it may be as effective as CR when it comes to improving overall health and potentially slowing the biological aging process.

A yearlong study of a hundred obese volunteers compared ADF to the standard CR practice (at 25 percent reduced calories). They found that both groups, in contrast to controls who maintained their normal eating habits, experienced 5 to 6 percent weight loss. There was a clear difference in adherence, however. Just under 40 percent of participants assigned to the ADF group quit before the study concluded, compared to just under 30 percent who were assigned to CR. This suggests that ADF may unfortunately be less sustainable for people in the long run—an important consideration, since these diets are only potentially effective if adopted as part of a healthy lifestyle. There is no long-lasting quick fix.

5:2 Diet

The 5:2 intermittent fasting diet is exactly what it sounds like. Each week, you fast for two days and eat normally for five. The diet shot into the spotlight thanks to enthusiasm from celebrities like Beyoncé, Benedict Cumberbatch, and Jimmy Kimmel. For instance, last year the famed late-night host reported that the diet had helped him lose significant weight but, more important, maintain the weight loss. As with FMD, the two fasting days of the 5:2 diet are not complete fasts, though there are some hard-core followers who do consume zero calories on the fasting days. Most people limit their food intake on fasting days to about 25 percent of their normal caloric needs. For the 5:2 diet, there are also no pre-specified days that the fast needs to fall on. This makes it much easier for people to fit it into their everyday lives. One could, in essence, rearrange a fasting day so that it doesn't coincide with a big social event or holiday. On most weeks, many people find it easier to space out their fasting days, allowing for two to three normal days of respite in between. While the exact food one eats on either the fasting days or the normal days in many ways is up to the individual, many try to stick to a plant-based diet (at least for the two fasting days), while others might follow a high-fat, low-carb diet.

The reason 5:2 has become so popular is because there is no entrance fee and very few hard-and-fast rules. This also means, however, that there is somewhat less scientific evidence to back the practice, as compared to the more regimented intermittent fasting diets, like FMD. If you are someone who is interested in trying 5:2, aside from consulting your physician, other considerations to keep in mind include the following: (1) You should attempt to eat nutrient-dense whole foods as much as possible, especially on fasting days. This will ensure you are getting the most from your food, including necessary vitamins and minerals to properly support your body. (2) The number of calories should be tailored to your activity level. While most people stick to 500 to 600 calories on fasting days, you may need to increase this if you are highly active on those days. I would not recommend running a 10k at the end of a 500-kcal fasting day. (3) The five "normal days" do not translate to binge days. For many people, the relief after a fast or anticipation of a fast may encourage overeating. Remember, it is important to also try to stick to as healthy a diet as possible on the off days if you want to maximize the benefits of fasting days.

Time-Restricted Eating (TRE)

Just like the name implies, this fasting practice is defined by restricted time windows in which you are allowed to eat. While not intentional, most of us already naturally fast for about eight hours a day while we sleep. It's no surprise that the first meal of our day is aptly named "breakfast." With TRE, however, the length of time between the last meal before bed and the first meal the next day is extended to somewhere between twelve and eighteen hours. For instance, some minimal TRE practitioners split their days in half, perhaps eating between seven a.m. and seven p.m. and then fasting at night. While it might not seem like much, this will often eliminate the late-night snacking that many of us are prone to and could be a good option for someone wanting to dip their toes into intermittent fasting before jumping in feetfirst. Often people doing TRE will extend their fast by simply skipping one of the regular meals of the day, typically breakfast. This may mean consuming your first meal at either noon or sometimes as late as two p.m. If the first meal of the day clocks in at noon or two p.m. and the final meal of the day clocks in around eight p.m., this equates to sixteen to eighteen hours of fasting every day.

For those who are even more extreme, the typical three meals per day plus snack may be collapsed into a single meal (often dinner). For example, Jack Dorsey, the founder of Twitter, was famously quoted as saying that he eats only once per day. What's more, he apparently combines TRE with 5:2 and consumes nothing over the weekend. Other celebrities who have allegedly jumped on the extreme TRE bandwagon include Pippa Middleton, Channing Tatum, and Herschel Walker. While celebrity endorsement should never be a reason to get behind a new diet trend, the data coming out of major research universities are starting to show TRE is more than a rapid weight loss fad. In a small pilot trial, researchers from the Salk Institute and the University of California, San Diego, showed that a three-month intervention in which subjects followed a ten-hour TRE protocol (i.e., eating during a ten-hour window and fasting fourteen hours) helped subjects shed abdominal fat, as well as improve blood pressure, cholesterol levels, decrease blood sugar, and increase insulin sensitivity.

EMPIRICAL BASIS FOR FASTING

Despite the fact that the practice of fasting dates back centuries, the science of fasting is still new. As such, there is still a lack of data comparing the various fasts head-to-head. While there is good evidence for each of them, we don't know what the ideal fasting time window should be. Some say twelve hours fasting and twelve eating (obviously not continuously), others say sixteen hours fasting and eight eating. Some people restrict to one meal a day, while others designate whole days to fasting. In the end, the ideal fasting regimen may end up being different for each of us. Given our different metabolic needs, fat stores, and physiological responses, the answer to "How long should you fast?" may be "It depends." Luckily, as our ability to estimate personal biological aging changes continues to improve, each of us will be able to empirically assess whether our nutritional abstinence is worth it.

Additionally, the fast that is best for you may just come down to which one you can actually maintain. For many of us, short-term fasts like TRE seem attainable. It's hard to fast for a whole day—or for that matter, multiple days. But most of us have enough willpower to put off eating for a few hours. What's more, many TRE enthusiasts report that their bodies adjust quickly, and they don't experience feelings of hunger until their typical eating window arrives.

That being said, personal preference will vary, and some people will prefer a few challenges a year, paired with normal eating the majority of the time. It is up to you to determine what works. If we compare fasts on the basis of the frequency one would do them versus the fasting time required by each, then FMD might be an option for people wanting something infrequent, but with longer fasting time (for example, five days). The 5:2 fast is in the middle for both duration (twenty-four hours of fasting) and frequency (only a few times a week), while TRE is daily (high frequency) but for a shorter bout of time (often twelve to twenty-three hours—approximately eight of which you are sleeping through).

But what is it about this historic practice that has such a profound impact on our bodies? While researchers are still trying to decipher all the effects of fasting, there are a number of things we have uncovered that may start pointing us in the right direction. Mostly, what it seems to come down to is a phenomenon called "hormesis."

Hormesis refers to a mild stressor that, rather than being detrimental, actually promotes a beneficial response in our bodies. Much like exercise, fasting appears to prime the body for repair and maintenance. It may signal to the body that food is scarce and thus chemical instructions are relayed to promote survival rather than use this time of deprivation to grow and/or adapt. Like with CR, the body is, in essence, turning off less essential processes and reverting resources to maintenance or repair. Things like IGF-1 signaling, which promotes growth, are dampened, and inflammation also tends to be dialed back. Some studies have even reported that our brains undergo transformation in response to prolonged fasting, promoting the generation of new brain cells and connections.

KETOSIS

One of the critical switches that occurs during a fast is the transition to different types of energy sources. When fasted, the body will often expend glucose and glycogen (the available blood sugar and its stored form). If those are exhausted, your metabolism then starts burning fat, which is the body's most concentrated energy source. This fat is converted to a chemical called a "ketone" that, because of its superior energy efficiency, is thought by many scientists to be protective of various age-related diseases. While there are no ideal systems, the closer your cells are to 100 percent energy efficiency, the slower your aging might be. Numerous studies have shown that ketones may help prevent development and growth of cancerous tumors, given that cancers rely heavily on forms of glucose (not ketones) to derive the energy needed for them to proliferate. Ketones have also been shown to reduce inflammatory processes and in turn are believed to protect against diseases like arthritis.

Given the central role ketones are presumed to play in eliciting the beneficial aging effects under fasted conditions, scientists and health advocates have asked whether one could initiate the switch to ketosis without having to withdraw food. The answer is yes! In fact, you may have already heard of the ever-popular keto diet, which does exactly that. By changing the proportions of macronutrients, individuals can force their body into ketosis while still enjoying (as my dad would call it) three squares a day.

The ketogenic diet only has a few simple rules, basically 5 to 10 percent of calories should come from carbohydrates, while the majority (about 70 percent) should come from fat, and the remainder from protein. Early adoptions of this diet in the 1920s were used mainly to treat children with epilepsy. At the end of the twentieth century, however, the low-carb diet trend helped keto gain in popularity as a means to lose weight. Recently, keto has also caught the attention of scientists studying aging, with the idea being that it may be a feasible CR or fasting mimetic, meaning it could induce the same beneficial effects without having to reduce calories. By limiting carbohydrates in the diet (the main source for glucose), one could force the body to switch over to using ketones as its primary energy source.

Studies from animals are showing that the keto diet may slow the rate of biological aging. For instance, mice put on the diet at about twelve months of age (considered middle age for a mouse) exhibited significant increases in life span and had molecular signatures that mirrored those observed under caloric restriction. What's more, a separate study by Dr. Vishwa "Deep" Dixit, a colleague of mine at Yale, showed that, like humans, older mice were at greater risk of dying over the course of the study and/or experiencing complications when infected with a mouse-specific strain of coronavirus, but that those on a ketogenic diet seemed somewhat protected. They had increased T cells (called "gamma delta T cells") that aided in protection and also showed less inflammatory response, which may make them less likely to experience the dreaded cytokine storm that has been linked to adverse outcomes.

While this starts to look like keto is the way to go if your goal is to slow aging, you might want to wait before stocking up on keto-friendly foods. Like most things, keto seems to be best in moderation. In a recent study published in *Nature Metabolism*, Dr. Dixit's team (the same group that showed keto may be beneficial for preventing serious complications from COVID-19) highlighted potential drawbacks of long-term keto adoption. While the protective gamma delta T cells will spread throughout the body and reduce inflammation and improve metabolic functioning after only a week, over time, fat consumption will outpace needs, leading to problems with breakdown and storage. Eventually, the protective T cells diminish, and metabolic problems and obesity dramatically spike, a condition called "ketosis."

Another issue with long-term ketosis is something called "ketoacidosis," which is when excessive ketones build up in the body, making blood levels dangerously acidic. While ketoacidosis is typically a condition that needs to be closely monitored in people with type 1 diabetes—given that they cannot produce insulin in order to lower ketone production—recently it has also been observed in long-term followers of the keto diet.

Finally, another danger is that, in order to meet the necessary macronutrient requirements of keto, most people end up consuming large amounts of meat and/or other animal products. If the goal is low carb and high fat, eating cheese, eggs, and steaks is a fairly easy way to ensure this. Conversely, many of the foods comprised by plant-based diets are off-limits—things like sweet potatoes, whole grains, and even many vegetables are too high in carbohydrates to work well within keto. As described earlier, animal-based, low-carbohydrate diets are linked to earlier death and higher rates of heart disease and cancers in humans.

Given all of the data to date, it seems that cycles of ketosis, as observed in intermittent fasting or short bouts of the keto diet (but with low animal-product intake), may be an effective method for slowing biological aging and improving overall health. Yet, despite the results coming out of studies looking into nutrition and aging, we have to remember that these generally reflect the average effects for all people (or animals) in the study. Within each of these studies we see variation—not everyone will respond in the same way to any given diet. While plant-based may be best for most people, that does not mean it is best for all people. Moreover, differences in genetics may dictate what macronutrient composition is best for each of us. Later on, in chapter 10, I will discuss how biological age measures can help you find what's best for you.

8

Exercise and Aging

If exercise were a drug, everyone would be clamoring to take it!

Physical activity exerts profound and lasting health benefits across various systems and organs in our bodies, from our bones to our hearts, and even our brains. No matter your age, disease status, or athletic proclivity, nearly everyone can benefit from staying active. Regular exercise has the ability to improve strength and balance, increase energy, reduce excess fat accumulation, improve mood, and even minimize stress. What's more, daily activity has been offered up as an additional explanation for longevity across the Blue Zones.

Unfortunately, the average person alive today only spends two hours per week engaged in physical activity. Yet this inactivity is in apparent opposition to the context under which our bodies evolved. In early human populations, physical activity was a daily endeavor. What we think of today as athletic capacity and strength was instrumental to survival. I often contemplate this while running in the rural Connecticut woods near my home, where bear sightings are a common occurrence. Luckily, I haven't had to put my speed and endurance to the test, but for most of human evolution, the world was a far more dangerous place than it is now.

THE NEED TO BE ACTIVE IS IN OUR DNA

Beyond avoiding being prey, physical ability enabled early humans to bolster their standing as major predators in the food chain. Back in the day, if you wanted a steak for dinner, you had to catch it first. Unfortunately, when it comes down to it, humans are slow. On the surface, we look like a pretty sorry excuse for a major predator. Eight-time Olympic gold medalist and world record holder Usain Bolt, who is considered the greatest sprinter of all time, would have a hard time chasing down any large (or even most small) herbivorous prey—if you have ever tried to catch a chicken, you know what I mean. In a quarter-mile race against an elite thoroughbred racehorse, Usain Bolt would barely be into the second turn when his equine competitor crossed the wire.

Yet science has revealed that the skeletal and muscular systems of humans actually evolved in a manner that appears specifically designed for running very long distances, and it is in this context that we can actually hold our own. To prove this point, for the last forty years, humans and horses have been lining up in the Welsh town of Llanwrtyd Wells to battle it out over the 22-mile track. In most years, the horses remain the victors; however, in both 2004 (Huw Lobb) and 2007 (Florian Holzinger), humans proved they can (at times) run faster than a racehorse. Physical endurance was key for our early ancestors, who would track prey for dozens of miles. Eventually, the animals would no longer be able to elude their human pursuers and, voilà, dinner.

Our bodies are conditioned to expect regular physical activity as part of daily life. But for too many of us, we spend the majority of our days sitting in chairs, driving in the car, or venturing twenty feet to the kitchen for our next meal. The vision of running dozens of miles to catch dinner has morphed into ducking out of the office during a brief break between meetings to grab a quick bite from the café around the corner. The result—dysregulated and declining physiology. A perfect example of "use it or lose it." Over time, continued inactivity causes our muscles to weaken, our hearts to be less efficient, our bones to be more brittle, and our agility and balance to waver. Everything we see in aging is only accelerated by lack of exercise. This also means, though, that we have tools at our disposal to offset these changes by altering our approaches to physical activity.

As with our ancestors, exertion should be a normal part of daily life, not an extracurricular activity. For many of us, this needs to be intentional. Our built environments promote sedentism, as most of us are tethered to a desk for the majority of our waking hours. This is detrimental to our aging process, and it has even been suggested that "sitting is the new smoking." For instance, findings from a 2011 study of nearly 800,000 people showed that those who reported sitting the most had a twofold increase in diabetes risk, a twofold increase in cardiovascular disease risk, and a 50 percent increased risk of early death compared to those who spent the least time sitting. This is bad news for many of us. Beyond investing in a treadmill desk, most people aren't willing to embark on a career change just to meet their stand goal for the day. Luckily, ensuring you get a moderate amount of exercise each day may be a powerful enough antidote.

EXERCISE AS AN ANTIDOTE FOR DISEASE

When it comes down to it, the effects of exercise on health and aging are remarkable. Numerous studies have pointed to the benefits of exercise for both disease management and disease prevention. It has been shown that interval training can reduce disease progression and increase life expectancy for individuals already diagnosed with heart disease and/or hypertension. Adoption of a regular exercise regimen has been shown to reverse type 2 diabetes, and among cancer survivors, physical activity has been linked to greater survival and lower risk of recurrence, particularly for breast cancer.

Perhaps the most powerful effect of exercise, however, appears to be its link to preventing disease altogether and, in turn, extending health-span. Empirical evidence suggests exercise can drastically reduce the immediate risk of nearly all major age-related diseases. Data suggest that exercise lowers the risk of up to thirteen different types of cancers. Regular physical activity has also been demonstrated to prevent the risk of developing Alzheimer's disease, a condition for which there is currently no treatment or pharmacological means to delay progression. Moreover, in 2012, researchers out of Harvard projected that lack of exercise within the population at large directly contributed to 5.3 million excess deaths in 2008. If true, this suggests widespread adoption of exercise could have prevented one of every ten deaths that year.

The reason exercise is such a potent strategy for preventing or delaying aging and disease is that it elicits a direct response in nearly every organ and system in our bodies. The temporary stress induced by physical activity will prompt various physiological adaptations aimed at boosting robustness, efficiency, and capacity. The goal of these is to prime your body so that it is better equipped to cope with a similar perturbation should it be encountered in the future. This is what makes living systems so amazing: they are adaptive. Unlike a car that can't adjust its functioning in order to meet demands, our bodies can. And by sending signals to our bodies to toughen up, we inevitability will improve resilience overall. To paraphrase German philosopher Friedrich Nietzsche, "What doesn't kill you makes you stronger."

PUMP IT UP

One of the most noteworthy adaptations to exercise occurs in the cardiovascular system, which is made up of the heart (cardio), the blood vessels (vascular), and of course the blood running through it. The main job of this system is to supply oxygen and nutrients throughout the body to be used to generate energy. Thus, it makes sense that cardiovascular output—or how much blood is being pumped around the body—can be dictated by the oxygen demands and uptake of working muscles during exertion. In the case of regular exercise, in which the system regularly encounters periods of high oxygen demand, your body will adapt and become more efficient. The lungs will increase their capacity to take in more oxygen with every breath. The heart will boost its ability to pump more blood throughout the body. Capillaries will amplify delivery of oxygen to muscles, and muscles will in turn put more oxygen to good use when it comes to generating energy.

The functioning of this system of oxygen consumption, delivery, and utilization can actually be measured using a variable called "VO2 max." VO2 max is measured by estimating how many millimeters of oxygen you consume over one minute, divided by your body weight in kilograms. While getting a precise measure of your current VO2 max typically requires a trip to the lab, where you will be hooked up to an expensive machine and asked to run at full exertion on a treadmill, there are also less cumbersome ways to acquire a rough estimate of your levels. According to the American Heart Association, one way is simply to determine how far you can run at full capacity over twelve minutes. Another, somewhat less strenuous method is to use a fitness tracker and combine information on heart rate and pace over a given time, say ten minutes.

While our VO2 max will naturally decline as we age, exercise can be an extremely effective means of offsetting this. For instance, a proven way to help maintain high levels of VO2 max is by engaging in regular aerobic exercises (running, biking, swimming), ideally with short durations performed at or near current VO2 max levels. Knowing your VO2 max and working to improve it is a critical part of maintaining health and well-being with aging. It will help you feel more energized throughout the day, and make routine challenges like climbing a flight of stairs, walking the dog, or playing with the grandkids much less strenuous and thus more enjoyable. As a bonus, data also suggest that it may help you stay disease-free for longer. A study tracking over 25,000 healthy middle-aged and older women in Norway showed that having a high VO2 max dramatically decreased the likelihood of having a heart attack over the fifteen-year follow-up. Similar results have been shown in large studies of men.

IGNITING YOUR ENERGY FACTORY

In addition to cardiovascular health, exercise also improves the functioning of other bodily systems that decline with age. For instance, not surprisingly, exercise has the capacity to reshape our metabolism. The most obvious way is that it helps burn excess energy, reducing blood sugar levels and depleting energy stores in adipose tissue. This explains why exercise is a powerful antidote for obesity and diabetes. Yet exercise also appears to improve your body's metabolic machinery. It has been reported that both the number and the size of mitochondria in our cells increase in response to regular physical activity.

If you recall, mitochondria are your body's powerhouse. They convert the nutrients you ingest into energy in the form of adenosine triphosphate (ATP). This converted energy can then be used by cells to go to work. Thus, the more numerous and more powerful your tiny factories are, the more efficient you become at generating usable energy. Additionally, exercise stimulates your body to be better at storing energy (glycogen) in skeletal muscles and to improve its capacity to utilize fat. Overall, this helps to deplete the unhealthy fat storage in adipose, while maintaining available energy for use in muscles.

These metabolic changes in muscle will also increase what is called "lactate threshold." When one exercises at high intensity, metabolism is revved up to meet energy needs. Unfortunately, this produces a by-product called "lactic acid," which you may have heard of. Many athletes regard it as the bane of their existence. This acid can create feelings of nausea, exhaustion, muscle cramping, and pain, most of the sensations that make many people hate exercising. Luckily, our bodies are also equipped to clear this acid, and with regular exercise, they become even better at it, explaining why running a mile for the first time in a decade may feel like torture, but after a few short weeks of training, it becomes a walk in the park.

Interesting new data from the Exercise Physiology Laboratory of Dr. George Brooks, a professor at UC Berkeley, suggest that not only does exercise boost the liver's ability to dispose of lactic acid, it may also help teach our muscle cells how to convert it for use as an energy source. When muscle cells use anaerobic metabolism to generate energy, they produce lactic acid. During very intense exercise, however, another metabolic pathway is ignited, called "oxidative aerobic metabolism." This pathway enables mitochondria to uptake, oxidize, and burn the accumulating lactic acid to produce even more energy. It may also explain why exercise boosts mitochondrial number and functioning and, in doing so, may prevent much of the biological aging that stems from mitochondrial loss and dysfunction. In fact, it has been said that exercise is the best medicine for promoting mitochondrial health.

EXERCISE AND THE IMMUNE SYSTEM

Both exercise and mitochondrial functioning also have important implications for the health of one of our most critical physiological networks, the immune system. With the emergence of COVID-19, many people have come to recognize just how important healthy immune functioning is. As was clearly demonstrated by the age-associated increases in

COVID-19 symptom severity, our immune systems tend to decline with aging. Systemic inflammation increases while our pathogen defenses begin to fail. The threat of COVID-19 actually prompted a number of people to reevaluate their behaviors and take steps toward improving their health. One way was through exercise. As reported by a large study out of the United Kingdom, a substantial number of older adults (those ages sixty-five and older) actually increased their levels of physical activity in response to the pandemic. Science tells us that this was likely a very smart move. In addition to getting in shape and feeling more energized, people probably increased their chances of survival if infected, since exercise has a substantial positive impact on a few key components of our immune system.

Immune response to viral or other infections comprises two phases: innate immunity and adaptive immunity. Briefly, the innate immune system is the first line of defense, the 911 response to an invading pathogen, foreign object, or injury. The distinction for this type of immunity is that the steps in this process are considered nonspecific, meaning that your body will mount a similar system of attack for anything that it identifies as foreign. Basically, something dangerous is detected and your body shoots first and asks questions later. The actions in this response are often orchestrated by proteins called "cytokines" (sometimes categorized as pro-inflammatory or anti-inflammatory cytokines). When a threat is identified, cytokines are expressed, which triggers an inflammatory response, recruiting and activating cells like macrophages and natural killer cells whose job it is to swiftly neutralize or destroy a threat before it can spread throughout the body. This highly active system underlies the increase in body temperature (or fever) that often accompanies an infection, or accounts for why heat and swelling are typically observed at sites of injury. Additionally, some cytokines, called "interferons," can act directly on cells to restrict viral replication.

The other arm of immunity, adaptive immunity, refers to the adaptations the immune system makes in response to a novel pathogenic stress:

fool me once, shame on you; fool me twice, shame on me. This learned or acquired immunity relies mostly on two types of cells: (1) B cells, which elicit antibody responses; and (2) T cells, which serve several supporting and primary roles. After maturing in the bone marrow, naive B cells (those which have not been exposed to an antigen) are released into the bloodstream, each with its own unique surface receptors that are able to bind specific antigens (i.e., surface markers found on various bacteria, viruses, fungi, or chemicals). If a B cell encounters and binds one of these antigens, with the help of a T cell it can essentially engulf the foreign object and break it down to make new receptors that are then placed on its surface. These B cells then generate clones of themselves (memory B cells), each with the same critical surface receptors. Some of the B cells will also transition into what's called a "plasma cell," which is able to pump antibodies into the bloodstream that can mark specific antigens for destruction. Like the surface receptors, these antibodies are able to bind the specific antigen that first initiated this sequence of events. Overall, this system is set up to enable the body to learn about potential foreign threats so that it can better guard against them should they be encountered again in the future.

T cells are the other critical component of adaptive immunity. Over a person's life span, the role of T cells changes. During early life, the system is mostly focused on developing immunity, while in adulthood, once immunity is mostly stable, the role of T cells shifts to maintaining homeostasis by regulating the response to common exposures and undergoing surveillance for aberrant cells, such as cancers. T cells can be classified into different types. As the name suggests, helper T cells help. They enable B cells to integrate information on pathogens and generate antibodies, and they also facilitate the ability of various immune cells to destroy pathogens. Conversely, the job of cytotoxic T cells is to kill the body's cells that have been infected by a virus before they can replicate, as well as cells that have turned cancerous or been irrevocably damaged.

Overall, the immune system is an amazing feat of engineering, but over time it begins to fail. Inflammation runs rampant as cytokine activation becomes dysregulated. This can elicit an overreaction in response to a pathogen, as is seen in the cytokine storm observed in COVID-19. Just like innocent civilian casualties or devastation to infrastructure that happens during a war, so too will cells and supporting tissue structures get caught in the cross fire. Another issue with a dysregulated innate immune response is that it can become chronically activated even when threats are not present. Aging is often associated with chronic low-grade inflammation. While a full-on war isn't taking place, something akin to a military occupation might be. This chronic inflammation is actually one of the most detrimental parts of immune aging and can predispose an individual to any number of diseases, including cancer, diabetes, heart disease, and rheumatoid arthritis. The adaptive immune system also begins to fail. The thymus—a specialized lymphoid organ located just behind your sternum that generates the naive T cells that are central to the adaptive immune response—drastically shrinks with age. This alteration, referred to as thymus involution, is thought to underlie the decline in immunosurveillance with age and the age-related increase in risk of infectious disease and cancer. B cells also lose function with aging, making vaccines less effective in the elderly while simultaneously increasing the propensity for autoimmunity.

Luckily, exercise is one thing that has a profound influence when it comes to combating these age-related changes in immune system functioning. Exercise activates a plethora of immune responses and overall leads to downregulation of inflammatory pathways. Numerous studies have demonstrated that both aerobic exercise and strength training can reduce signatures of inflammation in blood, muscle, and fat cells. The thymus also appears to respond to exercise. Physical activity can boost thymic output, as demonstrated by a study that looked at over one hundred long-distance cyclists in their fifties to eighties. Remarkably, what they found was that these individuals were able to maintain T cell production levels that were equivalent to levels observed in people in their twenties.

This observation, among others, may explain why physical activity protects against cancer and infection. Physical activity also seems to boost vaccine response in the elderly. Among those aged sixty-five and older, a significant proportion do not respond to vaccines, like the annual flu shot. This means that even though older adults get vaccinated, their bodies don't initiate an antibody response, leaving them susceptible to infection. This creates a major dilemma, given that these same individuals are often the ones most at risk of serious complications if infected with something like the flu virus. For this reason, vaccines for people over sixty-five are often altered to contain either a higher dose or an additive called "MF59 adjuvant," which initiates a stronger immune response. Exercise, however, can also help older adults elicit appropriate responses to vaccines. Studies have shown that antibodies were detected at higher levels following the flu vaccine among older adults who engaged in regular physical activity as compared to those who were sedentary.

EXERCISE AND YOUR BRAIN

While there are a number of direct health benefits that arise as a result of immune system responses to exercise, reductions in inflammation and improved immunity can also impact a number of other systems throughout the body, one of which may actually be the brain. Inflammation in the brain is thought to drive neurodegeneration and increase propensity for Alzheimer's disease. Two critical brain cells called "microglia" (which are the brain's immune cells) and "astrocytes" (which are the brain's support cells) have a propensity to become chronically "activated" with aging.

When this happens, it triggers the expression of pro-inflammatory cyto-kines and leads to sustained neuroinflammation. This toxic environment leads to functional and structural damage to neurons. Neuroinflammation is also thought to exacerbate the accumulation of plaques, which are one of the major hallmarks of Alzheimer's disease.

Another interesting immune-related link to brain aging is the hypothesis that Alzheimer's could be caused by germs. This idea, which was proposed decades ago and was long ignored by the inner circle of scientists working in the field, has recently emerged as a real possibility. By looking at thousands of postmortem brain samples, researchers began noticing an interesting pattern. The brains from people with Alzheimer's disease were more likely to be infected with viruses, particularly herpes simplex virus 1 (aka oral herpes). But how does a virus that remains mostly dormant and is known to infect the oral mucosa end up becoming activated in our brains? The answer—the aging immune system.

Yet perhaps one of the most striking demonstrations of how exercise can impact the brain was a 2020 paper published in *Science* by Dr. Saul Villeda's group at UCSF. Rather than exercising mice and then directly assessing the impact on their brains, the group actually administered the blood from exercised mice to non-exercised older mice and then looked to see what happened. They found that the process improved hippocampal functioning—the hippocampus is the critical region for learning and memory. The premise is based on the idea that exercise promotes the release of factors into the blood that have beneficial effects throughout the body, including in the brain. Thus, even if a mouse is not physically active itself, providing these factors could mimic the beneficial effects as if they were. Through this research, the scientists were also able to identify specific factors that may be responsible for this amazing finding. One of the factors, called "Gpld1," is expressed by the liver in response to exercise. They showed that administration of Gpld1 could improve cognitive performance in old mice. They also found higher levels of Gpld1 in the blood of healthy, active older humans.

IT'S NEVER TOO LATE

While breakthroughs like this suggest that perhaps one day we will be able to recapitulate the benefits of exercise with administration of factors like Gpld1, for now exercise still remains one of the best antiaging interventions "on the market." This is true even for the most frail among us. While the image of nursing home aerobics classes may not be the first thing that pops into our minds when we think about fitness and health, the science suggests that exercise isn't something people should undertake only when they are young, fit, and healthy. Rather, there doesn't seem to be an age in which the risks of being active outweigh the benefits. For many frail older adults, exercise is all too often viewed as something dangerous. Frail individuals are often worried that exercise may lead to falls or injury. Many view themselves, or are viewed by others, as too weak to partake in meaningful physical activity or can't imagine how activities that they are capable of will have any appreciable benefit on their condition. When we look at the data, though, we find that the opposite is actually true.

One of the major contributors of frailty with aging is called "sarcopenia." It refers to the progressive loss of skeletal muscle mass and strength with age and is thought to be a direct contributor to many of the physical impairments people suffer from in late life. Sarcopenia is what we refer to as a "multifactorial geriatric condition," given that it stems from myriad age-related changes reflecting alterations in hormone levels, declines in neurological functioning, increases in inflammation, escalating prevalence of insulin resistance and glucose intolerance, and growing propensity for fat infiltration in muscles. Sarcopenia is also a major risk factor in older individuals and substantially increases the risk of falls and/or fractures. This in turn can elevate an individual's likelihood of hospitalization or even death. Yet, while the drivers of this condition are many, currently there are only two interventions that reliably work to combat these changes—diet and, you guessed it, exercise!

For the past few decades, clinical trials in frail individuals (most with sarcopenia) consistently illustrate the benefit of both aerobic and strength/resistance training. Various small intervention studies have shown that monitored endurance training (often in the form of indoor cycling or walking) can improve peak VO2 max, which reflects both cardiovascular and lung health, and by itself is a strong predictor of future health risks. It also contributed to increased muscle mass in extremities, counteracting the effect of aging on sarcopenia. Not surprisingly, resistance training also appears to have a substantial impact on muscles in frail elderly. In a randomized control trial, scientists showed that among frail nursing home residents (often considered the most vulnerable population), ten weeks of resistance exercise training increased muscle strength by 113 percent. Walking speed, which is an indicator of physical and cognitive function, was increased by 11.8 percent; stair-climbing power, which captures muscle force, was increased by 28.4 percent; and thigh muscle mass, which can be a direct measure of sarcopenia, was increased by 2.7 percent. In the end, the authors of the study concluded that resistance exercise training is a viable and constructive means by which to counteract age-related declines in muscle mass and strength, and could improve physical functioning even in very elderly frail individuals.

In addition to sarcopenia, another degenerative condition that threatens our independence as we age is osteoporosis. Osteoporosis refers to the age-related loss of bone density and is characterized by porous, brittle bones. As a result, osteoporosis can greatly increase the risk of fractures with age. Bone is a living tissue that, like many other parts of our bodies, is continuously being broken down and replaced, and osteoporosis can occur in the face of excessive breakdown, impaired replacement of lost bone, or both. For most people, bone mass peaks around age thirty. As we age, the body's ability to generate new bone often can't keep pace with breakdown, resulting in progressive loss of bone density as we grow older.

This problem can be further exacerbated by hormonal changes with age, particularly in women, for whom declines in estrogen levels after menopause are seen as one of the biggest contributors to osteoporosis development. For this reason, hormone replacement therapy is often used to combat the risk of postmenopausal osteoporosis. Many of these therapies have been shown to improve the rate of bone turnover, helping preserve bone mineral density and reducing the risk of spine and hip fractures. But hormone replacement therapy is not without risks. For some women and at certain doses or durations, it can drastically increase the likelihood of developing breast cancer. Other medications for osteoporosis also exist, and while they have been successful in helping many people who suffer from this debilitating condition, like many drugs, they often come with unwanted side effects. Therefore, mitigating bone density loss through behavioral interventions, like exercise, is considered an ideal non-pharmacological intervention (often in addition to medication).

For individuals with osteoporosis, a routine involving regular exercises multiple times per week can go far to slow or prevent that rate of bone degeneration. One of the most common exercise routines that is recommended is strength training or resistance exercise, and in fact, the World Health Organization (WHO) recommends that individuals over the age of sixty-five should engage in muscle-strengthening activities no less than two days per week. These exercises involve the use of free weights, exercise bands, weight machines, medicine balls, or other forms of resistance and can be especially advantageous when targeting major muscle groups attached to the hips and spine. While the degree of intensity should be customized to an individual's ability and safety concerns, high mechanical load (lifting or pulling what feels like 80 to 85 percent maximum weight capacity) can stimulate bone remodeling. These activities will also improve muscle mass and strength, leading to greater stability and lessening the likelihood of falls.

THE IDEAL EXERCISE PRESCRIPTION

While all this data confirm the benefits of exercise, the numbers can be confusing when we try to evaluate what types and how much exercise we should be doing to get maximum benefit. As alluded to throughout this chapter, physical activity can take many different forms, even beyond distinguishing strength training from aerobic exercise. Even if routines that combine the two may provide the most benefit overall, your goals when it comes to offsetting various components of biological aging may also dictate what you focus on. While resistance training with weights may better serve individuals worried about declining bone and muscle health, aerobic exercises like running, biking, and swimming will have greater benefits for things like VO2 max. Relatedly, it isn't always clear how much and what level of intensity of exercise is optimal.

In general, the exact adaptations and responses your body elicits during exercise will vary as a function of things like exercise duration, intensity, physical force, and your baseline fitness level. Moreover, because the benefits of exercise stem from adaptations, that also means they can be fleeting. As with CR, exercise really needs to be maintained if you want to see long-term outcomes. Prolonged periods of inactivity, what is commonly referred to as "detraining," can undermine many of the benefits that were once gained. While it's great to be active during your youth, saying you were an athlete in high school or college isn't enough to rest your laurels on. It may prove beneficial in the short term, but having a big impact on aging will likely require a lifetime of consistent physical activity. In the end, it's important to find something you can stick with for the long haul. While spending an hour every day in the gym leading up to a high school reunion, wedding, or some other desirable end date may be a short-term solution, each person needs to evaluate whether a routine can be sustained within the constraints of their everyday lives.

For many of us, the biggest determinant of whether we exercise regularly comes down to time. With so many people in the workforce balancing long hours with commitments at home, finding that extra hour or more can be challenging. Even if we have a period of downtime during the day, many of us are exhausted and the last thing we may want to do is head to the gym for a prolonged sweat session. Luckily, evidence is emerging that one of the best exercise routines you can do doesn't take any more than thirty minutes. What's more, it is something you can undertake from the comfort of your home, without the need for fancy equipment, critical eyes, or a thirty-minute round-trip drive to your local fitness center. It's called "high-intensity interval training," or HIIT. In 2017, a study out of the Mayo Clinic showed that three months of HIIT was enough to substantially increase VO2 max. It also boosted mitochondrial functioning in muscle, and improved insulin sensitivity.

Generally, HIIT combines aerobic and weight-bearing exercises using very intense, short bursts of activity. For those of you familiar with exercise moves, think burpees. Each individual exercise performed during the approximately thirty-minute session is done for anywhere between thirty seconds to a minute and a half. The point is to go all out each time. Thus, HIIT is very different from a traditional cardio workout, like thirty minutes on the treadmill, in which someone is probably training at about 50 to 70 percent of their max heart rate. During HIIT, it is not uncommon to get your heart rate up to 90 percent of max during the short bursts and then letting it fall back to around 60 percent of max during brief rests in between. In many ways, the rest periods are as important as the exertion periods. They enable you to hit maximum output during intervals, help your body learn to recover faster, and force your system to adapt to cycling back and forth between stress and rest. Remember hormesis (low-dose stressor with beneficial physiological effects)? HIIT is a perfect example of it. The intensity of HIIT helps develop an adaptive stress response. When you are in a high-intensity interval, it temporarily throws your body out of homeostasis (your body's state of equilibrium defined by a specific temperature range, heart rate, chemical levels, and so on). Your body then needs to adapt to this perturbation by way of something called "allostasis," which is the body's physiological response in an effort to return to equilibrium or homeostasis. You throw your system off-kilter and it responds in order to restore balance (homeostasis, stressor, allostasis, return to homeostasis). Over time, these cycles of stress and response will make your body stronger and more resilient as it becomes primed and ready to offset and adapt to the brief deviations away from its normal state. Muscle fibers grow back thicker and denser, mitochondria become more efficient at generating usable energy, and processes like inflammation are turned down.

Given that the physiological stress induced by exercises like HIIT helps build a more robust body that is better able to cope with the unavoidable threats it will encounter day-to-day, one might think that more exercise would be even better. Interestingly, the data suggest it's not. That's because hormesis only works if it's brief, or what we call an "acute stressor." The converse—chronic or long-term stress—is actually detrimental. According to the *Merriam-Webster* dictionary, hormesis is defined as "a theoretical phenomenon of dose-response relationships in which something that produces harmful biological effects at moderate to high doses may produce beneficial effects at low doses." Basically, exercise is a stressor for our bodies—it contributes to muscle breakdown, puts strain on our cardiovascular system, requires tremendous energy output from our mitochondria, and even challenges our bodies' collective ability to regulate our temperature and dissipate heat. When the stress is manageable, it triggers our bodies to become more robust. Yet when the stress is too extreme or long-lasting, the benefit does not outweigh the cost. There is too much damage to repair or not enough time in between stressors in which to respond.

TOO MUCH OF A GOOD THING?

So where is the happy medium and how do we know how much is too much? While this is hard to study in the clinic, we are able to compare the aging and longevity trends of elite athletes or ultramarathoners to your average exerciser. In doing so, we are beginning to see that there is a U-shaped association between certain activities (like running) and health. What that means is that health risks (namely, cardiovascular events, diabetes, and even cancer) are highest for individuals who are sedentary, what some might call "couch potatoes." These risks fall for people who regularly engage in running moderate distances, say fifty miles a week over five days, but as the amount of running creeps up toward what we might consider extreme levels, the health risks begin to rise again. According to the data, it looks as if ultramarathoners actually have decreased healthspan and life span compared to "regular" runners. Essentially, there is a sweet spot that produces the greatest health benefits, which is good news for those of us with a full-time job and/or a family, who can't devote multiple hours a day to our runner's high.

Taken together, this suggests that, like Goldilocks, we need to figure out what type and amount of exercise is "just right." Just like diet, however, this is easier said than done. What might be "just right" for me may not be "just right" for you. A likely scenario is that we each start at a different baseline of stress tolerance. What is moderately stressful for one person's body may be very stressful for another's. Basically, exercise should be undertaken in accordance with the individual's current abilities, and each of us should slowly build up until we find our ideal sweet spot, whether that is running a 5k four times per week, taking Pilates reformer classes, doing daily walks around the neighborhood, or mixing it up and doing a little of everything.

As with diet, to some extent the types and amount of exercise that is best for you may come down to your personal characteristics, including genetics, experiences, health status, demographics, motivations, and what works with your lifestyle. Even if, for example, science tells you that HIIT may provide the greatest benefit for your health, if the only thing that works with your daily routine is thirty minutes on the elliptical three times a week, then do that. Finally, to optimize our exercise routine to produce the best net benefit for health, we will need to have well-established readouts (or biomarkers) of health and aging, like biological age. The ones available today are already powerful tools that give you a glimpse into your underlying biology and health, and in the future, the insight we can gain from these measures will only continue to grow.

The other thing to keep in mind is that the types and duration of exercise that might be ideal may not suit you overall. Exercise does not have to be vigorous or time-consuming in order to have a net positive benefit. In fact, numerous studies have shown that just thirty minutes of walking each day is enough to improve cardiovascular health, maintain muscle mass, and strengthen bones. Walking is great because it has a low bar to entry. It's free, doesn't require specific expertise, it isn't intimidating, and besides a decent pair of shoes, there is no special equipment. What's more, it can be done socially with friends, family, or pets, and in some cases, it can give us a chance to venture outdoors and perhaps take a moment to connect with nature.

Some of my favorite memories growing up in California are the hikes I would take with my family in the Santa Susana Mountains. The hilly terrain helped elevate my heart rate and stimulate my muscles. The time spent with my loved ones solidified lasting memories that I cherish today. And immersion in the amazing California landscape instilled my curiosity about nature and connections among all living things. Truth be told, these experiences were so precious to me that I still remember writing about them for my college admissions essay. And that's the point—exercise shouldn't feel like a chore, it should be enjoyable. The key is to find something you love doing, whether it's basketball at the YMCA, walking your dog, going to Pilates with friends, or riding bikes with your kids. As Michelle Obama's campaign urged, "Let's Move." These days, my weekly exercise comes in the form of horseback riding, which I currently do five days a week. Although I had been a runner and athlete growing up, once I hit adulthood, and especially after I became a mom, I found it harder and harder to maintain my routine of daily runs, gym classes, and/or exercise videos in my living room. While I still participate in these from time to time, I have had more success in treating exercise like a pastime rather than a prescription.

9

Rest and Relaxation

Diet and exercise are the king and queen of health behaviors. There are a number of other actions, however, that can define a healthy or unhealthy lifestyle. While I won't cover things like smoking which have obvious and non-debatable impact on overall health, factors like sleep, stress, and socioeconomic characteristics have also been shown to have profound impacts on aging, life expectancy, and health in general.

THE POWER OF SLEEP

Whenever I find myself critically evaluating my lifestyle to determine where improvements can be made, the category that repeatedly rises to the top is sleep. As with many busy professionals, I constantly find that there aren't enough hours in the day to get everything done. With work, family obligations, and hobbies, I often end up trying to catch up on work late into the night, only to have my alarm go off early the next morning. Even on nights that I'm in bed at a reasonable hour, I have a tendency to lie awake mulling over my schedule for the next day, or fixating on exciting research questions that pop into my head. Suffice to say, I rarely get more than seven hours of sleep a night and I am lucky if I even get that.

I realize this may have a negative impact on my health and, as such, is something I am constantly striving to address. Like the other health behaviors we have discussed, sleep can impact functioning across your many body systems. There is one system in particular, though, that is especially impacted by sleep: the nervous system, or more specifically, the brain. To understand this, perhaps we should start by discussing why sleep evolved.

We humans spend more than a quarter to a third of our lives asleep. If you are lucky enough to survive to age one hundred, that means you've been asleep for a total of twenty-five to thirty years. What's more, going without sleep can be lethal. Studies have shown that rodents can die after only two weeks of sleep deprivation.

The other, perhaps paradoxical, evidence supporting the importance of sleep is that sleep is dangerous, or at least it was for early humans and most animals in the wild. When you are sleeping, you become vulnerable. Your senses are diminished, and your brain is in many ways "offline." You suddenly become easy pickings for a hungry predator. If sleep did not have a critical role to play in our health and evolutionary fitness, this trait would have never been selected for.

So, what is so important about sleep? What is happening behind our closed eyes that elicits such profound impacts on our health to offset the risks it also incurs? While the truth is that nobody really knows, science is starting to uncover some of the physiological changes that take place while we are getting our ZZZs, and many of them are quite remarkable.

Like most parents, I have found that convincing a five-year-old that it's time to go to bed is a challenge like no other. She wants to play. She wants to chat. Despite being too full to finish dinner only an hour ago, she is suddenly ravenous, or parched, or needs to use the bathroom for the sixth time tonight. About a year ago, I decided to try a different tack, and started trying to explain to her why she needs to go to sleep. I don't tell her it's because I need time to work, or just frankly need a moment to myself. I tell her it's because sleep helps to "clean her brain." While this tactic isn't foolproof, it has helped my life each night. In fact, some mornings she is even concerned whether I had enough sleep to clean my dirty brain. Luckily, my daughter has inherited my type A tendencies, and the idea of a dirty brain is something that must be remedied. What I've explained to her is that while she sleeps, her body actually washes out all the dirty things that accumulated in her brain over the previous day. While this sounds silly, it is actually based on new evidence that has been cropping up from scientific studies on the neuroscience of sleep.

WHAT HAPPENS BEHIND CLOSED EYES

Within our spinal cords resides a clear liquid called "cerebrospinal fluid," or CSF for short. CSF is very similar to the plasma in blood, except that it contains far fewer proteins (about 0.3 percent of those in plasma). CSF is also almost entirely cell-free, meaning you won't find any red blood cells and it contains very few white blood cells. CSF has many roles in the brain. For instance, it keeps the brain buoyant. The weight of our brain bearing down on itself would cut off blood supply and cause massive damage if it weren't suspended in liquid CSF. Similarly, CSF also provides a buffer for the brain in case of impact and, like blood, CSF helps transport nutrients and other chemicals around the brain. One of CSF's most fascinating roles, however, is its ability to clear waste or damaged factors from the brain during a specific phase in our sleep cycle.

Overall, there are two main types of sleep—rapid eye movement (REM) and non-REM. During the night, our bodies transition through sleep cycles involving three stages of non-REM followed by one stage of REM sleep. These cycles each last around ninety minutes, meaning that you will experience approximately four to six of them on any given night. (As an aside: sleep cycles tend to last only forty minutes for newborns, and their inability to reliably transition between cycles on their own can lead to the plaguing sleep deprivation experienced by many new parents.)

Sleep cycles always begin with the first stage of non-REM sleep which, as one might imagine, is characterized by the transition period between wakefulness and sleep. Everything begins to relax during this phase; but because this sleep stage is very light, it can easily be disrupted by noises or movement. After a few minutes in stage 1, sleep will give way to the second stage when everything slows down. This is the most frequent of the four cycles if you were to add up the total time spent in each throughout an entire night. During stage 2, body temperature drops, heart rate slows, muscles relax, breathing becomes shallower, and brain activity dampens.

After about twenty to forty minutes in stage 2, there will be a gradual transition to stage 3, what is considered deep sleep. During deep sleep, your body will relax even further and go "offline." As such, it takes a lot more to awaken someone during deep sleep. Brain activity will also change during this phase. The neurons in our brain communicate with one another via electrical pulse, and during deep sleep, these pulses take on a different frequency denoted by shortwave activity patterns (around 1.5 to 4 hertz). Early in the night, you will spend more time in stage 3.

As the night goes on and eventually transitions to morning, stage 3 will become shorter and shorter. Conversely, the last stage of sleep, called REM sleep, is truncated during the first few cycles, lasting maybe ten or twenty minutes. The amount of time spent in REM becomes progressively longer with each subsequent sleep cycle, however, and eventually may encompass the majority of the cycle as morning approaches. REM is thought to be the active form of sleep, when vivid dreams occur. Temporary paralysis sets in to prevent your body from acting out the scenes of your dreams, yet your eyes begin to move rapidly, hence the name. Brain activity is more reflective of what is seen during wakefulness, and your heart rate and blood pressure move closer to normal levels.

REM and non-REM both seem to be important when it comes to memory consolidation. They help ensure that important memories from the day are converted into long-term storage, while inconsequential ones are left to fall by the wayside. Yet the two forms of sleep are also believed to play specific roles in health. Overall, REM sleep seems to be important when it comes to improving mental and emotional health. While it is not clear if the benefits of REM sleep are a direct result of dreaming or something else, studies have shown that it may help stress processing. It's been shown that getting more REM sleep may dampen the negative reactivity experienced by individuals with post-traumatic stress disorder (PTSD). It's also been shown that getting more REM sleep the night before a traumatic event can make it less distressing. REM also seems to play a role in emotional intelligence, helping us judge facial expressions, read emotions, and process these external stimuli—and perhaps not surprisingly, lack of REM sleep can leave a person feeling irritable the next day. As a result of these impacts of REM on emotional and mental well-being, some researchers have likened this stage of sleep to a nighttime therapy session.

Deep sleep, by contrast, seems to be the major player when it comes to the physical revitalization we associate with sleep. It's the restorative form of sleep when muscles repair themselves, collagen is replaced in skin, and insulin and glucose levels are restabilized. During this phase, nonessential processes are also downregulated so that energy can be allocated toward maintenance and repair. In recent years, scientists have discovered fascinating new ways in which deep sleep impacts our health. One of these is the brain cleaning that I brought up previously.

Remarkably, emerging evidence suggests that the process of clearing waste from our brains is driven in part by the shortwave oscillations, called "delta waves," that manifest during deep sleep. While we have known about delta waves for more than a century, we are only starting to discover how these frequencies may coordinate the removal of waste from our brains.

SLEEP AND BRAIN REJUVENATION

During sleep, but not during wakefulness, very large waves of CSF can be observed washing over our brains. By combining electroencephalography (EEG) with a functional magnetic resonance imaging (fMRI) technique, a team of scientists from Boston University and Harvard were able to observe blood flow, CSF flow, and electrical activity simultaneously. What they discovered was that the oscillations of delta waves were in sync with the swell of CSF. The slow rolling electrical brain activity was cyclically changing the volume of blood flow through vessels. When constricted, this would make way for CSF to fill ventricles and the subarachnoid space that surrounds the brain matter. Unlike blood, CSF can also flow directly into the brain tissue, bathing brain cells before being absorbed back into blood vessels through which it exits the nervous system. What's more, the CSF that flows through our spinal cord and brain cavity is continuously replaced every eight hours, essentially providing a clean bath to wash away new debris.

Since this remarkable function of CSF was first discovered, scientists have wondered whether this bathing of our brains has implications for neurodegenerative diseases like Alzheimer's. As previously mentioned, in Alzheimer's, brains often accumulate two hallmarks called "amyloid beta plaques" and "neurofibrillary tangles." One hypothesis is that CSF is actively working to clear these potentially toxic factors away and this ability is further enhanced by the delta wave oscillations that occur during deep sleep. While sleep disturbances are a common complaint in individuals with Alzheimer's disease, data are mounting that the link between neurodegeneration and problematic sleep may be more than a symptom. Sleep problems may actually drive disease progression. Studies are showing that disrupting sleep or stimulating excitatory neurons that control arousal promote the accumulation of various Alzheimer's markers in mice. Similarly, sleep deprivation seems to do the same to humans. This can create a compounding effect if ailments of aging, including cognitive ones, cause sleep disturbances, which in turn further drive degenerative declines.

HOW MUCH SHUT-EYE?

Despite this chicken-or-egg scenario, it is clear that sleep, particularly non-REM deep sleep, plays a critical role in our health as we age. But again, that doesn't mean that more is always better. In fact, like exercise, the link between sleep duration and outcomes of health is U-shaped. The optimal level actually centers somewhere around seven hours a night. A huge analysis, looking at sleep data across sixteen unique studies on nearly 1.4 million people, showed that short sleep duration, which was defined as less than five hours per night, was associated with a reduction in life span. It was actually prolonged sleep, however, that exhibited the biggest risk of death over the course of the study. What's more, the longer the sleep, the more the risks increased—that is, there was a slight increase for those getting an average of more than eight hours, a bit larger increased risk for those getting more than nine hours, and the biggest increase in risk for those getting ten or more hours each night. This trend also seemed to hold regardless of a person's age, gender, or socioeconomic status.

As with many observational or epidemiological studies, this association is not indisputable proof that lack of sleep or excess sleep will decrease your life expectancy. The causal direction of this association has not been substantiated. Many disease conditions, like depression, thyroid problems, heart diseases, and sleep apnea, can contribute to oversleeping. In these cases, it is not clear whether it is the condition itself that confers the increase in mortality risk or whether excess sleep is further contributing. To make things even more complicated, many scientists have argued that it is not necessarily sleep quantity that matters, but rather sleep quality.

My friend Julia is serious when it comes to her sleep. She does everything right. She makes sure to get outside in natural sunlight each day. She reduces her blue light exposure at night by staying off the computer after nine p.m., limiting TV watching, and not scrolling through her phone. She never consumes caffeine past two in the afternoon. She doesn't snack on anything after dinner, and she makes sure her bedroom is conducive to getting shut-eye by turning the thermostat down to 65 degrees each night. At ten p.m., she promptly climbs into bed and enjoys thirty minutes to an hour of her current audiobook before falling asleep to the echo of crashing waves on her sound machine. Then every day at six a.m., she awakens to her sunrise alarm clock that fills her bedroom with glorious dawn-tinted streaks of artificial sunlight.

Sounds ideal, right? Not quite. Unfortunately, Julia feels compelled to undertake this elaborate sleep ritual because her sleep is anything but ideal. As a mother to a young child, she is constantly woken and often has a hard time falling back asleep. To make matters worse, her partner is what Julia calls "a division 1 snorer." Just as she starts to drift back to sleep, a loud snort jolts her awake. Often this can continue for what feels like hours, and as the clock progressively continues to tick toward morning, Julia becomes more and more stressed about all the sleep she is missing. Not only will she likely feel tired and irritable at breakfast, but as a public health researcher, she knows that sleep disruptions can impact her health.

QUANTITY VERSUS QUALITY

This comes back to the relative importance of the different sleep stages. Waking up and losing out on deep sleep or REM can make you feel like you spent less time in bed even if you got a full seven or eight hours. That's because every time you fully wake up, you start back at the beginning, leading to a decline in the amount of deep sleep you may be getting. In two studies on the links between sleep and health, researchers found that the quality of one's sleep was more strongly related to things like mood, fatigue, and depression than sleep quantity. What's more, in 2018, I was a part of a study that examined the links between epigenetic aging and sleep in a cohort of women.

The main author on that paper, Dr. Judith Carroll, found that differences in the amount of sleep was not associated with our aging outcome. Participants seem to have similar epigenetic aging regardless of whether they reported sleeping an average of five hours or nine hours. We did observe major differences, however, as a function of what Dr. Carroll defined as "insomnia symptoms." These referred to frequent experiences of restlessness, waking in the night, trouble falling back to sleep, and early awakenings. The more of these issues women reported having, the older they appeared on an epigenetic level, regardless of what their chronological age was. Moreover, women who reported insomnia symptoms also appeared to have worse immune functioning. One caveat is that similar to the links between sleep duration and health, we could not conclude in this study whether sleep disturbances were *causing* accelerated aging or whether accelerated aging was impairing sleep. In fact, the latter makes scientific sense, given that problematic sleep may signal disruptions in the body's internal clock.

Within each of us is an internal clock, referred to as "circadian rhythm," that plays a crucial role in regulating the cyclical patterns of various physiological functions. It is how our bodies keep time. Circadian rhythm is a twenty-four-hour clock that dictates things like sleep or wakefulness, the release of hormones throughout the day, changes in body temperature, cellular regeneration and turnover, and even metabolic processes. Because this biological clock has such sweeping implications for nearly every physiological function in our body, disruption to the cycle can have major health implications.

Similar circadian clocks are thought to operate in nearly all living organisms, including other animals, tiny microbes, and even plants. This is rather amazing, as you can imagine, since twenty-four hours for us is a lifetime for some species. It's believed that circadian rhythm evolved in accordance with geological phenomena, in that it is tuned to the environmental changes that occur as a function of the Earth's movement—mainly changes in light. Basically, living systems evolved a remarkable technique for tracking time as a function of the Earth's rotation (i.e., days). In contrast to a mechanical clock that ticks out time using cogs, gears, and springs, our biological clock is regulated by the oscillating changes in expression of specific genes. At the core of this timepiece are two genes, one aptly named CLOCK (circadian locomotor output cycles kaput), and the other BMAL1. Together, the expressions of these two genes elicit the perpetually cycling changes observed in circadian rhythm via their effects on the epigenome. By modifying the epigenetic landscape, these factors alter the accessibility of various gene components, turning them on or off and thus contributing to the oscillations observed in circadian rhythms.

Another gene that has been shown to be critical to this process is SIRT1. This is noteworthy because SIRT1 is the human version of a gene called SIR2. As I mentioned earlier, in 1999, Dr. Leonard Guarente, along with two young colleagues—Matt Kaeberlein and Mitch McVey—showed that overexpression of SIR2 had antiaging mechanisms and could extend the life span of yeast by as much as 70 percent. Numerous other studies out of the Guarente lab, made by Dr. David Sinclair and others around the same time, further demonstrated the importance of SIR2 for regulating the epigenome and maintaining genomic stability over the replicative life span of a yeast cell. While you may rightfully argue that humans and yeast cells are very different, there is some data to suggest that the effects of SIR2/SIRT1 may be evolutionarily conserved. That means the same pathways through which SIR2 regulates the life span of a yeast may be operable for regulating our life span. Even in mice, slight overexpression of SIRT1 has been shown by some researchers to protect against cancer, senescence, oxidative stress, and DNA damage.

Some scientists are also positing changes in SIRT1 expression are responsible for the beneficial effects of caloric restriction. Basically, they are saying that CR only increases life span because it boosts SIRT1 expression. Thus, without the SIRT1 increase, there would be no longevity gain for going hungry. While there is debate in the field as to whether that effect is true, SIRT1 has been shown to be a major metabolic sensor in our tissues. Based on environmental cues, modulation of SIRT1 expression can cause epigenetic changes that in turn alter tissue processes including stress response, energy metabolism, remodeling of fat tissue, and inflammation.

SIRT1 also offers an exciting link between aging, metabolism, and sleep. Using genetic or pharmaceutical manipulations, scientists have shown that, in addition to the processes mentioned above, inhibiting SIRT1 can disrupt circadian rhythm. Unfortunately, declines in SIRT1 function naturally occur with aging, potentially accounting for some of the circadian deficits that are observed as we grow older. The decline in SIRT1 function occurs because of a loss of bioavailable NAD. As mentioned previously, NAD is needed for SIRT1 to function. Thus, as levels of NAD naturally decrease with age, SIRT1 becomes less effective. In

2013, Guarente's lab showed that these age-related declines in NAD-dependent SIRT1 activity in the brains of mice contributed to an elongated circadian clock (basically a longer day according to the animal's internal biological clock). These animals also exhibited disrupted activity patterns and difficulty in adapting to changes in light/dark oscillation (for example, the old mice would have had a much harder time coping with jet lag). Luckily, though, it was shown that the age-related effects could be counteracted by overexpressing SIRT1 in the old animals. Stay tuned—the story linking SIRT1, NAD, and circadian rhythm continues. In addition to SIRT1 levels eliciting effects on circadian rhythm, it appears that expression of circadian genes also stimulates the pathway that leads to increased NAD synthesis. This is one example of how disruptions in this pathway—due to natural aging, sleep disorders, or asynchronous sleep schedules—can have a snowballing effect on health.

One of the clearer examples of this comes from observations of night-shift workers. In modern societies, it isn't uncommon for individuals to spend nights working and then catch up on sleep during daylight hours. Unfortunately, this is not how our bodies are naturally set up to function, and this disruption to circadian rhythm can have negative health effects. In a randomized control trial, a group of young adults was asked to spend a week at a research lab. These study participants were then randomly assigned to two conditions such that half of them slept during the night and the other half slept during the day (similar to what a night worker would do). The research team collected blood samples from participants every three hours and then compared the two groups to identify changes in cyclical patterns of hormones such as melatonin and cortisol, as well as hundreds of metabolites.

What they found was that oscillations in melatonin and cortisol that are naturally seen in humans were unchanged in the two groups, suggesting that the internal circadian clock had not shifted to reflect the twelve-hour shift in sleep timing. This was not the case, however, for a number of metabolites that relate to liver, pancreatic, and digestive tracks. These all showed a twelve-hour shift in their cycles. The problem with this outcome is that the internal clocks of different organs became asynchronous. While the brain was signaling that it was nighttime, the body was signaling that it was day. This shift in metabolic processes versus nervous system processes may explain why individuals who work night shifts are often more prone to conditions like obesity and diabetes.

EXHAUSTING THE OPTIONS

For these individuals, improving health via better sleeping habits probably requires a complete lifestyle shift—which unfortunately may not be an option. But what are the options for people who suffer from insomnia or sleep disorders that are not due to their daily schedule? While diet and exercise feel much more within our control, sleep is one place where even the most diligent health nut can still struggle. Often, we find that the more we try to sleep, the harder it is to simply drift off. What's more, difficulty falling asleep can also be coupled with difficulty staying asleep—leading to poor sleep quality characterized by a lot of wakeful nights and unpleasant mornings.

For people who suffer from insomnia, the first solution they may reach for are over-the-counter sleep aids, and melatonin is one of the most popular. Briefly, melatonin is a hormone produced in your brain in response to low light, helping to regulate circadian rhythm. Essentially, your brain is signaling that it's nighttime and your body should prepare to wind down. This natural response to light/dark cycles is also one of the reasons many researchers and doctors encourage low lighting and reduced screen time in the few hours preceding bed. By mirroring the light changes outdoors, we can better ensure that our bodies are generating the correct circadian responses. Beyond this, oral supplementation or skin patch administration of melatonin can be used to bolster this signaling process. Often these will be engineered to allow for controlled release of the hormone into your bloodstream so that it can mimic the natural rise that occurs at night.

This is often not as simple a solution as it may seem, however. Our bodies can quickly adjust to melatonin supplementation, rendering it less effective within a relatively short time. As such, this type of sleep aid is usually recommended only for occasional use, such as helping you get to sleep during a stressful time in your life and/or in response to major circadian clock disruptions, like jet lag. Melatonin supplementation is not a cure-all for insomnia. The same goes for other sleep aids like doxylamine (Unisom and Sleep Aid) and diphenhydramine (things like Benadryl and Aleve PM). These two common sleep aids are composed of antihistamines that act via sedative effects, and thus often leave you feeling groggy the next day.

When it comes to melatonin, according to both the American Academy of Sleep Medicine and the American College of Physicians, there is not enough empirical evidence yet to support its use for treating chronic insomnia. In fact, both these organizations instead recommend a drug-free solution, what is called "cognitive behavioral therapy for insomnia" (CBT-I). CBT-I has repeatedly come up as one of the best treatments for insomnia, including conditions arising as a result of stress or PTSD. In a large meta-analysis of 181 unique studies on interventions to address insomnia disorders, CBT-I was the clear winner. It improved outcomes for all the sleep parameters examined, and also appeared to work across the board, from young adults to old adults, those with pain, chronic conditions, and the like. The best part is that unlike many supplements or medications, there are no adverse side effects of something like CBT-I. So why do more people reach for the pills when there is clearly a better solution?

For many, one of the incentives for turning to supplements to address sleep issues, rather than taking advantage of solutions like CBT-I, is that ordering a ten-dollar bottle of pills off the internet seems a lot simpler than trying to navigate our health system to receive treatment. For many people unfamiliar with CBT, they may hold misconceptions that this type of treatment involves Freudian-based psychoanalysis or sentimental discussions about getting in touch with your feelings. But in reality, CBT is based on a strong scientific foundation, shown to address numerous mental (and even physical) conditions. What's more, delivery of CBT has kept up with the times. You don't have to find a local sleep therapist or figure out where and how to book an appointment to receive CBT-I treatment. There's now an app(s) for that! One of these apps, called the Insomnia Coach, was created by the U.S. Department of Veterans Affairs' National Center for PTSD. Freely available to all, it provides a five-week training plan with tips, tracking (which can be assisted via wearable devices), and access to a sleep coach. Other apps, like CBT-i Coach, can be used to facilitate treatment options for those who prefer to work directly with a CBT-I provider.

In addition to directly training good sleep habits, therapies like CBT may also address a root cause of many individuals' sleep problems—stress! The link between stress and insomnia has never been more apparent than it has in recent years. With the disruptions in people's daily lives brought on by the global COVID-19 pandemic, more and more people began reporting problems falling and/or staying asleep. This became so prevalent that scientists and health experts started referring to it as "coronasomnia." According to a study out of the National Institutes of Health, people in the United States reported substantial increases in rates of clinically significant insomnia, coupled with higher rates of reported stress, depression, and anxiety. While isolated instances of stress and anxiety are bound to afflict us all, it is the chronic, long-standing instances of stress that have the potential to significantly disrupt aspects of our health, including sleep.

THE IMPACT OF MENTAL STRESS

As discussed previously in this book, acute mild stressors can be beneficial to our health. They can often challenge our systems, helping them toughen up. Continuously repeated stressors (or what we call "chronic stress," like those experienced day-to-day), however, can eventually wear us down. Stress can be physical, as in the case of physically demanding labor or prolonged malnutrition. But for many of us, it's psychological stress that plagues us. According to the National Institute of Mental Health, more than a third of us experience continuous anxiety, and millions present with depression-related disorders each year. And it's no wonder. Our modern world breeds stress. We are constantly on the go, playing catch-up and hardly ever feeling like we have a handle on everything we need to get done. Our lives are much more publicly scrutinized than ever before. We have very little alone or quiet time to just sit and reflect. Our work culture promotes competition and makes us very aware of our social and economic standing. Even if it seems that we are thriving and successful, it's hard to relax our pace for fear that we could lose it all at any moment.

Decades ago, it was suggested that the longevity advantage enjoyed by women stemmed from the fact that they were less likely to be in the workforce and thus did not have to deal with the job stresses that plagued men. Based on this assumption, some warned that if women entered the workforce, they would be increasing their stress levels and thus diminishing their health and happiness. The boom in career women over the last half century has painted a different picture, though. According to research out of Max Planck Institute for Demographic Research, women who took on careers actually seem to be doing better. By tracking the profession status and health of over 5,000 women for thirty-six years, the researchers observed that those who continuously worked experienced less decline in physical health as they aged compared to women who did not work outside the home. The women also reported having fewer depressive symptoms, suggesting that the stresses of work may have not had a major negative impact on their mental health.

The findings of this study should not be taken to suggest that work is always psychologically beneficial. Keep in mind that these are population averages and we each have our own unique set of personal preferences and constraints. For some, work may provide an outlet for creativity and self-fulfillment, while for others, balancing the expectations of work and family life may be overwhelming. This may be especially true for those with very little support either in their jobs or at home.

Starting in the 1950s, women's labor force participation began to steadily rise. In the United States, this grew from just under 35 percent to a peak of 60 percent by the turn of the twenty-first century. The wage gap has also narrowed, although not enough. Women have received more college degrees than men, and in 49 percent of households, women report being the main breadwinner. This was the case in my house growing up. My mother was a college professor who was in many ways the sole earner in my family. Yet, for the most recent generations, the rate of female workforce participation has somewhat receded. This was further compounded by COVID-19, which dealt a major blow, forcing four times as many women as men to drop out of the labor force during the summer of 2020.

One explanation for the leaking of female workers from the career pipeline is that despite women working more than their mothers' and grandmothers' generations, they were not getting a break at home. Despite the progress we have made, women still carry the majority of the burden when it comes to housework, raising children, and caring for ailing parents (even their in-laws). In fact, according to surveys, women spend an average of nearly one and a half hours per day doing household chores, such as cooking, cleaning, and doing laundry. This is compared to only thirty minutes reported by men on average. Furthermore, this doesn't seem to be a result of inequitable balance between couples, where perhaps the partner who earns less or has a less demanding career ends up doing more at home. This imbalance seems to have grown out of gender stereotypes. For instance, in same-sex couples, research has shown that divisions of labor at home are much more equitable.

This piling-on of responsibilities can cause major feelings of anxiety and even depression in female professionals. When comparing stress levels, women are more likely than men to report experiencing both emotional and physical symptoms of stress. This includes upset stomach, headaches, and feeling as though you are on the verge of crying. One interesting point is that married women seem to report even more stress than single women. Paradoxically, this is in stark contrast to the statistics reporting that, for men, marriage tends to be beneficial for overall health.

The solution for all of this is not to keep women out of the workforce or suggest that they should not get married and have children. Rather, as a society we need to figure out how to redistribute responsibilities so that the weight isn't concentrated on a subset of the population. This means recognizing and working to overcome our implicit biases regarding gender roles. Governments can also work to provide better social programs to help support individuals and families so that those who want to work (or need to work) have more support in other facets of their lives.

While these changes would go a long way toward ameliorating stress for women and men alike, there is another problem to contend with that can contribute to poor mental and physical health for women or other marginalized groups, especially in the workplace—a phenomenon called "stereotype threat."

As a society, we have implicit biases regarding the attributes of various social or demographic groups. Negative stereotypes can cause performance anxiety and doubts in the minds of individuals who belong to those groups. Ironically, subconscious apprehensions about confirming the stereotype can lead to a temporary deficit in cognitive ability, making it more likely that the individual will actually live up to it. This is called "stereotype threat" and it has been a long-standing focus of investigation in social psychology. One of the clearest examples of this relates to the stereotype that people of color and/or females are bad at math and/or perform worse academically. Reminding these groups of this stereotype before they take a test can actually cause them to perform worse.

A similar reaction happens in older adults undergoing a cognitive assessment. If a psychiatrist discusses how aging is a risk factor for dementia before they start the assessment, the patients will be more likely to exhibit a cognitive deficit. Similar dynamics are also at play in the workplace, especially in high-status or male-dominated positions. Individuals from underrepresented groups are implicitly conditioned to think that the reason there are fewer people like them in those roles is that they are not good at them. They second-guess their own leadership and negotiation skills, their analytical and tactical abilities. In the end, all this does is generate anxiety, fear, and self-loathing, leading to a self-fulfilling prophecy.

Stereotype threat is also closely related to another stress-inducing condition—imposter syndrome, although there is some evidence that this condition is easier to generalize and may not disproportionately impact marginalized groups. To demonstrate what it is, imagine for a moment that you get contacted by a major TV network which wants to feature you on their show. They say their choice is due to your expertise and amazing accomplishments. In the episode, they would like you to describe how you came to be so successful and to convey to others what they should do so that they can follow in your footsteps. They state unequivocally that your presence will truly be an inspiration to so many people in your field of work.

After you hang up the phone, your first reaction might be a feeling of pride and flattery. You have worked hard to get where you are, and it feels great to be recognized for that. For most of us, however, those feelings will quickly give way to doubt and insecurity. You ask yourself, "Why me? I can't really be the best choice for this role! Aren't there more deserving people out there, and if so, will this finally expose me for what I am—an imposter?" This all-too-common reaction is called "imposter syndrome." While the example I gave was an extreme scenario, imposter syndrome affects most of us on a continuous basis. Whenever we are asked to engage in a performance-based task, there it is, waiting in the wings.

There is an epidemic of imposter syndrome in academia and other high-stress jobs. It is unfortunately something I see constantly in myself and many of the PhD students I work with at Yale. Despite being extremely intelligent and high-achieving young adults, for many of them, imposter syndrome can be debilitating. It prevents them from making progress in their research for fear of not living up to the high expectations they set for themselves. They are all too often scared to ask for help for fear that it signals failure, and for too many promising young scientists, it can actually derail their careers. Yet even if they are able to recognize and battle through it, the stress associated with these feelings can manifest as major anxiety, low self-esteem, and even major depression.

THE MIND-BODY CONNECTION

The stress and anxiety associated with conditions like imposter syndrome, difficulties with work/life balance, and just the constant pressure experienced by so many living in this day and age, can impact more than just our mental health. In fact, the reason I am discussing mental health in a book about biological aging is because what happens in our brain directly connects to physiology in the rest of our body. In the face of psychosocial stressors, your brain will activate what is called the "HPA axis." This refers to the connections among three structures—the hypothalamus (a small structure at the base of your brain), the pituitary gland (a pea-shaped gland just under the hypothalamus), and the adrenal glands (small hormone-producing glands situated just over your kidneys). First, the hypothalamus releases a hormone called "corticotropin" that then tells the anterior pituitary to release an adrenocorticotropic hormone, which finally stimulates the release of a steroid hormone from the adrenal cortex called "cortisol."

While these names may seem hard to keep straight, the important part is the notion that stress activates the HPA axis and the end result is increased cortisol levels, the body's primary stress hormone. Cortisol has many roles in the body, including being a critical regulator of the fight-or-flight response. In stressful situations, cortisol can initiate the release of glucose into the bloodstream so that it is immediately available for use as energy in case you need to run or fight. It will shut down nonessential functions like digestion, growth, reproduction, and immune functions. And although cortisol gets a bad rep, its actions aren't innately bad. In fact, it was critical to human survival. But in the world in which the reaction of the HPA axis and cortisol release evolved, stresses were fleeting. They would happen and then just as quickly dissipate, allowing the body to return to normal—or homeostasis. By contrast, in today's world, most of our stresses are continuous. They don't let up, and therefore neither does our body's stress response. Over time, the sustained levels of elevated cortisol can wear down our system and increase risk of things like metabolic syndrome and diabetes.

A condition called Cushing's disease, first discovered by the famous neurosurgeon Dr. Harvey Williams Cushing in the early 1900s, illustrates the physiological effects of high cortisol levels. In Cushing's disease, there is an overabundance of cortisol due to an excess release of adrenocorticotropic hormone from the anterior pituitary, in most cases due to the presence of a pituitary tumor. Generally, cortisol levels follow a circadian pattern and are regulated by our circadian clock. They are highest in the morning and then drop throughout the day. In individuals with Cushing's disease, however, cortisol tends to sustain the high morning levels and doesn't show the expected diurnal dip. Common symptoms of these chronically high levels of cortisol include weight gain, fatigue, high blood pressure, and insulin resistance (diabetes), among others. Although Cushing's disease does not manifest as a result of stress, it does provide some insights into the potential risks associated with dysfunctional cortisol secretion.

Researchers have also observed that individuals under continuous stress will experience less dramatic drops in morning cortisol levels, observed as a flattening of the diurnal slope. This in essence means that cortisol secretion is not getting shut off when it is supposed to. One potential concern with this is that it may actually dampen the beneficial effects of cortisol. Again, cortisol is not all bad. It is a natural anti-inflammatory, much like the closely related hormone cortisone, which is often injected into joints to relieve inflammation and reduce pain. But when cortisol doesn't follow its normal up-and-down pattern throughout the day, your body may develop resistance to it, similar to insulin resistance in the case of diabetes. Your system is, in essence, crying wolf.

In one of Aesop's Fables, "The Boy Who Cried Wolf," the young shepherd decides to play a trick on the villagers who live nearby. He repeatedly calls out that there is a wolf in the vicinity. After so many times of reacting only to find there is no wolf in sight, the villagers stop responding to the boy's cries. Then one day, a wolf truly does show up. But this time, when the boy sounds the alarm, no one pays any attention. Needless to say, it doesn't end well—in the original version, only the innocent sheep lose their lives, but in later English adaptations, so does the puckish boy.

Back to physiology. In addition to its basic circadian functions, cortisol evolved to spike when there was an immediate stress or danger. Your brain would sense a threat and the HPA axis would be turned on to help you survive. Shortly after, everything would resolve, and things would go back to normal. In the case of psychosocial stress, however, the resolution never comes. Your brain continues to cry out, "There's a threat! We need to react!" but for the most part, these threats are not imminent dangers. As it was with the boy, your system becomes dulled to these spikes, and then when it's needed, cortisol is no longer able to do the things like decrease inflammation, regulate circadian metabolism, or even turn itself off.

In addition to the HPA axis, other connected brain pathways can further alter physiology in response to stress. For instance, the sympathetic nervous system (SNS) is one of three components of the autonomic nervous system, which directs the subconscious reactions and responses throughout our body. The SNS, specifically, is in charge of our natural fight-or-flight response. When you experience something stressful, you don't then say to your body, "All right . . . I need to elevate my heart rate so that more blood is flowing, dilate my pupils so I can see better in dim light, tense up my muscles so that they can better withstand force, and elevate my breathing so that I can take in more oxygen in case I need to run!" That is something your SNS will take care of for you. Scientists, however, including my colleague Dr. Steve Cole from UCLA, are also uncovering what happens when SNS stays on—as is often the case during chronic stress. Specifically, this has been shown to have substantial effects on our immune system.

The impact on immunity may not come as a huge surprise. We have all probably attributed the sudden emergence of cold symptoms at one time or another to "being run-down," and there is merit to this sentiment. SNS activity can impact the expansion of white blood cell populations. This does not happen equally across all white blood cell types, though, and there is a tendency for the body to expand its number of cells involved in inflammation—at the expense of those involved in antibody or antiviral response.

After observing this pattern repeatedly in response to a variety of psychosocial stressors, Dr. Cole coined the term "conserved transcriptional response to adversity," or CTRA for short. Similar to the other

SNS-activated changes like blood pressure, vision, and so on, this stress response profile is thought to have evolved to help us survive acute threats. For example, inflammation is critical in the case of an injury. So if there is a chance that you may have to tangle with a tiger, once the dust settles you better hope your body is also ready to fight anything that may make its way in through an open wound. In contrast, viral infections are typically only a problem when you are in social settings in which communicable pathogens can be passed from one person to another. Thus, our ability to protect against this threat is generally less important than running for our lives and is, therefore, suppressed by our natural stress response.

HOW TO COPE

Despite the fact that this response was a beneficial adaptation, meant to help us stay healthy and survive, in today's world where stress is rooted in our continuous daily circumstances, the constant activation of CTRA may promote inflammation, contributing to a spectrum of diseases like Alzheimer's, diabetes, cardiovascular disease, cancer, and inflammatory diseases. So what's the solution? We can't all quit our jobs and our family responsibilities and take up residence in an oceanside Zen oasis. Nor would we all want to. In fact, many of us can and do thrive off the stresses that consume our daily lives. It may just come down to perspective.

According to research by Dr. Alia Crum, a Stanford University psychology professor and the principal investigator of the Stanford Mind & Body Lab, embracing stress has the potential to make us smarter, healthier, and even happier. Her work has shown that those of us who view stress as a helpful part of life, or a challenge we welcome and are eager to overcome, end up better off because of it. Luckily, this seems to hold even in times of very high stress. Dr. Crum suggests that our perceptions of a stress can alter our response to it. Perceiving a stress as problematic can lead to negative reactions—whether it's coping via engagement in unhealthy behaviors, or attempting to avoid the stress, both of which increase risks for long-term outcomes like depression or other medical conditions.

Further building on the work by Dr. Crum, a fellow Stanford psychologist, Dr. Kelly McGonigal, a health psychologist and lecturer at Stanford, describes three beliefs that she states are the most beneficial ways to think about stress. First, she says that it is critical to regard the stress response as productive rather than crippling. While I have described a lot of problematic things that occur in response to stress, remember that these responses are beneficially adaptive. They are meant to provide you energy to deal with whatever major risk you are facing. If you use that energy to overcome a stressor, it will be much more beneficial than wallowing in it.

The second thing is to make sure to regard yourself as capable of overcoming the stressor. This idea harkens back to much of what we have learned from cognitive research about growth mindset. If you see yourself as able to grow and learn through dedication and hard work, you will be more likely to succeed than those who see their abilities as fixed.

Finally, it's important to acknowledge that stress is something that we all deal with. You are not alone in feeling overwhelmed or exhausted. In this same vein, our society also needs to reframe how we think about psychotherapy and mental health. We are all encouraged to visit our physician to care for our physical health. There is no reason why we shouldn't do the same for our mental health.

Similar to the benefits that exercise can bestow on our bodies, skills like mindfulness and meditation can improve our emotional well-being and tolerance to psychological stress. According to a randomized clinical trial headed by researchers at Carnegie Mellon University, those who engage in mindfulness training can reduce perceptions of stress. Through this training, participants were taught to bring about awareness of their present state without judgment. They also received instruction on attention to breathing, body sensation, and how to engage in basic activities like walking or eating from a mindful perspective. Similar to the three techniques described by Dr. McGonigal, mindfulness training can help individuals accept their current situation and grow from it. And this may be the key to blocking the negative effects of stress: science is showing us that how we perceive the stress in our lives may be more important to our health and aging than the events themselves . . . to an extent.

DISPARITIES AND
THE UNEQUAL DISTRIBUTION OF STRESS

For those of us who encounter stress due to highly competitive work environments, basic child rearing responsibilities, daily obligations, or personal expectations, those experiences can also come with rewards. Yes, we don't always see them as equitable, but there is at least an upside to these high-stress situations. That, however, is not the case for everyone. For many people, the major source of stress in their lives is from external sources far beyond their control. It's what we call "exogenous stress." While health can be impacted by a variety of circumstances throughout life, we all vary in the degree of control we have over these occurrences. As with genetics, some of us are simply born into circumstances with the potential to shape our entire aging trajectory.

On a shady tree-lined street in the Forest Hills neighborhood of Washington, D.C., sits a traditional brick colonial. It's centered by a cobblestone walkway, lined with a neat boxwood hedge with giant white hydrangea blooms that spill over the top of it during the summer months.

It is the home of the Fosters, who have just welcomed their second son, Daniel. On weekends, Daniel accompanies his family in his baby carrier as they walk through their quiet neighborhood, passing by the Embassy of the Kingdom of the Netherlands and the Hillwood Estate, Museum & Gardens (a thirteen-acre eighteenth-century-style estate, housing French decorative and Russian Imperial art). Often, they will visit Soapstone Valley Park, where Daniel's brother will run down the wooded trails, hopping across the stepping-stones of the creek, as other Forest Hill residents hike and run past.

Meanwhile, about twenty minutes south, across the river from the U.S. Capitol, the Davis family has just celebrated the birth of their son, James. The Davises live on the second floor of a cottage-style duplex in the historic Anacostia neighborhood. Anacostia is one of the oldest neighborhoods in D.C., home to Cedar Hill, an estate formerly owned by Frederick Douglass in 1877. A quarter mile down W Street SE from Cedar Hill sits another, more whimsical landmark—the Big Chair, an art installation designed in 1959 by the Bassett Furniture company. While it no longer holds the title of the world's largest chair, the twenty-foot structure stands amid a backdrop of a busy urban parking lot on the corner of Martin Luther King Jr. Avenue and V Street SE.

Unfortunately, while the longevity of Anacostia's most famous landmarks is notable, the same cannot be said for its residents. In fact, the median life expectancy is only around sixty-three years for a child like James. Meanwhile, in Forest Hills, the median life expectancy for Daniel is estimated to be just over ninety years. While James has a fifty-fifty chance that he will even live long enough to collect Social Security, Daniel is expected to collect his share for nearly two and a half decades (assuming the program remains solvent).

Forest Hills and Anacostia represent the juxtaposition that seems to exist throughout the world—and especially in the United States: two boys, both born in the same major metropolitan city in one of the richest countries in the world, yet having completely different outlooks when it comes to their life span and healthspan. This is because the zip code you live in is a major determinant of aging. People living just a few bus stops away can have dramatically different opportunities for longevity and health. Since discovering this conundrum, researchers have been hard at work trying to discover what it is about a place that can so strongly dictate our future.

There is a growing body of evidence highlighting the various links between poor health and living within what is categorized as a disadvantaged community. Such neighborhoods are traditionally places with high poverty rates, coupled with less access to adequate health care and services, high crime rates, increased air and/or noise pollution, and lack of recreational areas. Many of these locations are also what we call "food deserts," which are defined as geographic areas with limited to no access to affordable and healthy food options. This primarily refers to restricted availability of fresh fruits and vegetables. For instance, around 2 percent of households in the United States (some 2.3 million people) live more than a mile away from the nearest supermarket and do not have access to a vehicle. Recent data have also shown us that there are three times as many grocery stores in wealthy areas compared to poor ones. Even when grocery stores are present, in many low-income or urban neighborhoods they can be overshadowed by the vast number of fast-food restaurants that provide very affordable and quick meals. For individuals struggling to make ends meet, and perhaps working more than one job, an easy and cheap meal is hard to overlook.

The uneven distribution of food deserts across high- versus low-income communities points to how health behaviors can be shaped by disadvantage. Yet beyond the discrepancies in lifestyle, socioeconomic status also has a profound impact on stress. Decades of social science research, much of it led by my former mentor, Dr. Eileen Crimmins, has documented the health disparities between the rich and the poor, especially when it comes to aging. The data overwhelmingly suggest that one of the major culprits is stress. The constant fear that you may not be able to provide adequate food, shelter, or other necessities for yourself and/or your loved ones leads to chronic anxiety and stress. Millions of families across the United States face hunger and food insecurity every day, and the fear of not knowing if or when your next meal will come can in many ways be more damaging than the hunger pangs that accompany it.

Safe and affordable housing is another anxiety-ridden concern. In the United States in 2017, 2.6 million households with children and 1.9 million elderly households lived in what is deemed "worst-case housing needs," defined as a family with extreme rent burden, low income, and no government housing assistance. These families are at constant risk of losing their homes and joining the over half a million other citizens forced to live on the streets. While the stereotype of homelessness is often associated with substance abuse, the truth is that a large proportion of the homeless population is families—many single mothers and their children who cannot afford rent even with a full-time job at current minimum wage levels. What's more, even individuals who can afford rent or who receive supplemental assistance from the government are often forced to reside in less than ideal shelters or in areas with high crime rates, where they are saddled with constant fear for their own safety.

The compounding effects of the constraints and threats that plague the lives of low-income individuals lead to profoundly accelerated aging rates in these populations. For instance, we found that adversity and low socioeconomic status in adulthood accounted for nearly 12 percent of the differences in biological aging rates between individuals. This was the case while also considering the effects of health behaviors, demographics, and genetics (which ironically accounted for far less of the variance in aging). In that same paper, we define socioeconomic status and adversity as constraints that are beyond one's control. While some may argue that through hard work and dedication, one can better their situation—after all that's what the American Dream promises—the truth is, like most things it is not that simple.

According to new research from the World Economic Forum, most countries fall drastically short when it comes to providing the paths and opportunities that allow their citizens to thrive. This presents a major hindrance to social mobility, and in most cases an individual's socioeconomic prospects are anchored by the social class they were born into. As a result, the socioeconomic disparities, and the health discrepancies tied to them, can last for generations. In many countries, this comes back to geographic and neighborhood differences. Poor children have less access to good early childhood education. They experience repeated hardships as their families struggle to put food on the table and keep a roof over their heads. Their families can't afford tutors or SAT prep classes, or extensive extracurricular activities that seem to be a prerequisite to getting into a good university. Not to mention the cost of tuition, which presents a major roadblock for many families. Even if they do have the opportunity to attend university, stereotype threat and stress/anxiety, among other things, can jeopardize their performance.

Yet in spite of whether an individual is socially mobile (some people are clearly able to pull themselves up by their bootstraps), the adversity one is born into can have lasting and damaging effects on health. Sociologists Dr. Mark Hayward and Dr. Bridget Gorman refer to this as "the long arm of childhood." Early life experiences have lasting effects on stress signaling and health outcomes across the life course. Adverse childhood experiences (ACEs), including low socioeconomic status (SES), maltreatment, or maladaptive early-family environments, are associated with a broad spectrum of subsequent health problems in adulthood, including cardiovascular disorders (CVDs), metabolic abnormalities, cancers, arthritis, and mental illnesses. Evidence from both animal and human studies continue to point to chronic stress-induced inflammation as a central biological mechanism linking early adversity to aging and disease. Numerous studies, including some of mine, show that low childhood SES and harsh early-family environments are associated with elevated concentrations of inflammatory markers decades later, independent of the individual's current social standing.

CRITICAL PERIODS

The scientific investigation into adversity and stress during developmental stages of life have highlighted the concepts of "critical periods" and "biological programming." These theories suggest that unfavorable environmental circumstances during specific periods of development can program biological systems in a manner that persists across a person's life span and accentuates one's vulnerability to disease. For example, studies of early-life social exposures have shown that neonatal rodents that are handled daily exhibit diminished physiological responses to stressful experience when they reach adulthood. These developmental switches have been hypothesized to be the result of epigenetic processes that can alter the molecular responses when confronted with certain situations. From an evolutionary standpoint, this is how our system was programmed to be able to adapt to the world around us. In some cases, though, our body doesn't get it right and these adaptations can actually be detrimental to our long-term health.

One well-studied example of maladaptive epigenetic reprogramming during critical developmental periods is the example of the Dutch Hunger Winter (or *Hongerwinter*) during World War II. Starting in the summer of 1944, the German blockade cut off the food and supply chain to the Nazi-occupied Netherlands, leaving much of the country to go hungry. By the time the liberation of the Dutch people finally arrived in May 1945, it was reported that around 18,000 people had died from starvation. Like much of the events during that time, this tragedy brought with it profound suffering and loss, yet it also provided some scientific hints into how events in our history can shape our biology. Some forty-odd years later, epidemiologist Dr. David Barker stumbled upon an interesting observation arising from this natural (yet unfortunate) human experiment. Not surprisingly, he observed that women who were pregnant and in the mid- to late-gestational stages during the famine gave birth to babies that weighed significantly less than average, while those in early gestation had normal-sized babies.

But what was surprising was what would become of the "normal" babies. According to the data, those whose mothers were in the early stages of pregnancy during the Dutch Hunger Winter were far more likely to grow up to be obese when compared to the individuals born either before or after them. Later evidence would also show that this cohort was more likely to experience heart disease or other cardiometabolic conditions as they aged. Dr. Barker hypothesized that the epigenetic adaptations to food scarcity during critical developmental periods could become maladaptive when the situation changes. Once food is again plentiful, the body may still act as though it is not, thus leading to fat accumulation and its associated health risks.

A similar mechanism is thought to occur with psychological stress. Chronic exposure to stress and anxiety during development may prime physiological responses like inflammation, making individuals more biologically reactive to future stressful events experienced throughout life. As such, one can imagine how social and economic inequality can manifest enormous disparities in healthspan and life span.

RACIAL DIFFERENCES IN STRESS EXPOSURE

Perhaps nowhere is this more clear than when looking at the disease and mortality risks experienced by African Americans and/or other marginalized groups. In 2014, I conducted a study with Dr. Eileen Crimmins that compared the aging rates of individuals as a function of race. Years of epidemiological research has shown that Black people are on average more likely to experience disease and death at much younger ages than white people. Our hypothesis was that this was due to an acceleration of the aging process. What we found was that, when applying a measure of biological age, African Americans were on average three years older biologically than whites of the same chronological age. What's more, we showed that this entirely explained the disparities in mortality risk, cardiovascular disease, and cancer. While these conclusions may be misconstrued by some to suggest that there are innate differences by race, what was truly underlying these patterns was adversity.

Issues already discussed in this chapter, like socioeconomic status, neighborhood conditions, availability of health care, and repeated exposure to psychosocial stress, are all at play when it comes to generating the racial disparities we observed in our data. Science suggests that over time, these circumstances have the ability to get "under the skin," mostly through neurological stress response, alterations in hormone levels, or immune and inflammatory processes. Because Black people are also more prone to experiencing discrimination and stereotype threat, this can lead to further anxiety, with the potential to stimulate a plethora of biological changes that drive aging. In 1992, Dr. Arline Geronimus described her theory that the health and physiological functioning of Black individuals begins to deteriorate early in adulthood as a result of the constant and accumulating exposure to adverse outcomes over their lives. This concept, referred to as the "weathering hypothesis," has since been extensively studied in relation to socioeconomic and racial/ethnic health disparities research.

While there are clearly enormous strides that need to be made by our civic and government leaders when it comes to reducing economic disparities, improving social mobility, providing support for individuals and families, and working to improve mental health, science has also shown us that the human body is resilient. There is potential for improved health even for the most disadvantaged—some might say *especially* for the most disadvantaged. Again, most of the trends and statistics I have described in this chapter relate to group averages or generalizable patterns. This book is about personalization, however, and as such, it is important to remember that substantial variation underlies these data. Not everyone who experiences disadvantage or trauma should expect to die earlier, nor can those blessed with advantages rest on their laurels. Data on biological aging and disparities have shown us that there are clearly resilient individuals—those among us who can be knocked down by life, yet get back up and carry on stronger than before. What's more, there are likely things each of us can do in our own lives to bolster our fortitude against life's unfortunate surprises.

10

Finding Your "Just Right"

I n the nineteenth-century fairy tale "Goldilocks and the Three Bears," a young girl enters a house where she is met with various choices of where to sit, what to eat, and eventually where to rest her head. In each of these decisions, she tries out the various options, finally settling on the ones that are "just right." When it comes to biological age, I have thus far described how one could actually assess and track it, as well as the many facets of our lives that we think will impact it. I have described various diets, exercise routines, and mental health practices that are predicted to slow or even reverse biological age. But aside from my personal preference, I have not conveyed how you go about selecting what actions will be the most beneficial for you.

I will say that on some level, the answer is a bit disappointing . . . for now. Science has yet to discover a way to predict an ideal course of action. Researchers have tried to identify genetic differences between people that might provide clues, but as with most complex genetic traits, the results are far from predictive. We are currently working to discover epigenetic signatures that may uncover things like optimal diet or exercise for an individual, or determine whether a person may be more prone to deleterious effects from things like smoking, obesity, and/or drinking. Preliminarily, it does appear that your epigenetic signature may contain important insights into the potential effects of different behaviors. Enormous amounts of data, however, will be needed before these predictions can actually be used to help people make personalized decisions.

BECOMING YOUR OWN SCIENTIST

Armed with the insights biological age measures can provide, what's a person to do? How do you determine whether calorie restriction (CR), a plant-based diet, intermittent fasting, cyclical keto, or some combination is right for you? One option—start testing! While not technically a well-controlled study, tracking your own biological age can help you biohack your own aging process. In fact, there are people already doing this with seemingly great success. Reddit groups, like Blood_Testing_Aging, have cropped up with the goal of helping share tips on "Using blood testing to minimize disease risk, and to maximize health and longevity." Recently, a physician in the United Kingdom, Dr. Oliver Zolman, developed an "Age Reduction Leaderboard" on his website, which ranks individuals who have submitted data based on the difference in their chronological age and biological age. At the time I am writing this, Dr. Zolman himself is the top contender, with a difference of nearly seventeen years between his two ages (biological age being lower). Close on his heels is James Clement, at age sixty-five chronologically and forty-nine and a half biologically. James Clement is the president of Betterhumans, a scientific nonprofit organization focused on the biology of aging. He is also the author of *The Switch*, a 2019 book focused on the benefits of intermittent fasting, protein cycling, and keto, in which he describes the diet he has used to produce his over fifteen-year biological age deficit.

Another top contender is Dr. Michael Lustgarten, who at age forty-seven and a half chronologically, has a biological age around thirty-five. Dr. Lustgarten is a scientist at the Human Nutrition Research Center on Aging at Tufts University in Boston, Massachusetts. While all three men have a day job that relates to the science of aging, they don't have any secret information that has helped them stay young. No cutting-edge treatments or pills. Instead, they have used good old-fashioned health behaviors, coupled with real-time tracking of their aging to garner their way into the upper echelons of elite agers.

Over the years, Dr. Lustgarten has developed multiple blogs, videos, and social media groups chronicling his experiences using biological age measures to optimize his diet, exercise, and other behaviors. Like me, he believes that the pace at which we age is something that can be impacted by our behaviors and that slowing it has the potential to minimize disease risk and maximize health. As a result, Dr. Lustgarten has been actively tracking his lab tests for nearly two decades. Starting in 2003, he began entering all his annual or biannual blood test data into an Excel file. In 2015, he took this to the next level by increasing the frequency of testing to every two months and tracking the weight and macro- and micronutrients of all the food he consumed. Eventually, he used this rich personalized data set to help him select a diet that he felt produced the strongest benefit when it came to levels of his circulating biomarkers. He looked for correlations between his changing diet and individual biomarkers, to help him identify what potentially could be incorporated to bring them closer to youthful levels, and/or the levels associated with the greatest life expectancy.

A few years later, I published my phenotypic age measure and Dr. Lustgarten began to use the output to further optimize his tracking. At this point in time, his first phenotypic age measurement was 36.2 years, which was ten years younger than his chronological age. Since then, he has continued to measure his phenotypic age (he has currently measured it nine times and counting as of this writing). Despite the fact that his chronological age increases every year—as it does for all of us—Dr. Lustgarten has maintained a phenotypic age averaging just under thirty-five years and reaching as low as 32.9 years during his most recent test. He believes that this achievement was a direct result of his diet, which is composed of high beta-carotene-rich foods and at least 100 grams of fiber per day, mostly in the form of vegetables like carrots, broccoli, cauliflower, red bell peppers, spinach, and beets. This dwarfs the typical fiber intake for most people, which in the United States averages only about 15 grams per day. In addition to diet, Dr. Lustgarten has also made exercise a big part of his lifestyle, but he doesn't overdo it. He generally engages in about seven to ten hours of moderate/intense exercise each week—a mix of cardio and strength training.

For people starting out on this journey, Dr. Lustgarten suggests focusing on eating "real food" and improving fitness. He notes that the investment he has put in is extremely time-consuming and truly hopes that in the future, implementation of AI will help personalize diet, exercise, and supplements routines. Yet, for now, he will keep doing what he is doing in order to meet his lofty goal to "live longer than everyone that has ever lived." He notes that he doesn't have a family history of longevity, but he is determined to use "every bit of science . . . to at least live as long as [his] genetics allow, which is the best that [he] can do."

THE FUTURE IS NOW!

Most people don't have goals as lofty as Dr. Lustgarten's, nor the patience and dedication to do what he has done to try to optimize aging.

That doesn't mean that we can't do anything, though. We can all make small improvements in our daily lives that will likely translate into more disease-free years. The task is figuring out what is feasible for each of us and whether it is worth the time and investment.

Last month, my thirty-six-year-old, seemingly healthy husband went in to get a physical from his primary care doctor. During the appointment, he asked his doctor if he could get a referral for the lab tests used in my phenotypic age measure. His doctor was perplexed. My husband had nothing apparently wrong with him. He is a healthy young man who eats well and exercises regularly. His pulse and blood pressure were ideal. In his doctor's mind, there was no reason for him to request the lab tests. Both my husband and I track our aging, however, and make adjustments to our lifestyle in response. Eventually, she acquiesced, and he received the referral for the blood panel. Not surprisingly, when I crunched his numbers, he looked great—on the lower end of biological age for his birth cohort—but there was still room for improvement. My husband is an avid Apple Watch user and had a nearly three-year streak of meeting his move goal. He noticed, though, that he has been doing the same routine for so long that perhaps his body had adjusted. His heart rate didn't get elevated as much as it once did, and perhaps he was not getting the hormetic stress benefit that exercise once provided to him. He changed things up and six months later saw this reflected in improvements to his biological age. While we can't say with certainty what this did for his prospective healthspan and life span, it is an example how, even among young adults, actionable steps can be taken and tracked to slow aging long before disease symptoms ever arise. It's the first step toward optimization.

In addition to providing positive feedback, biological age tracking can also tell us when things are not working. Or perhaps more important, what things are not worth the time or investment (monetary or otherwise). For instance, dietary supplements are often touted as able to promote health and even slow aging. Currently there are more than 50,000 different supplement products on the market, which has become an over $40 billion industry. In the United States, however, unlike pharmaceuticals, supplements fall under the category of food and are therefore not held to stringent regulatory standards by the FDA. Companies are essentially free to make claims about their products' abilities to improve health without needing rigorous clinical trial testing. In fact, one of the only restrictions is that they cannot claim that a supplement can cure or treat a specific disease. Often these unregulated supplements can be dangerous. A 2015 paper published in the *New England Journal of Medicine* showed that approximately 23,000 emergency department visits in the United States each year were due to adverse reactions to dietary supplements. Yet even for those companies who follow protocols and standards to ensure safety, how are consumers able to determine whether they are actually getting the health boost being promised on the label or in ads? For the most part, consumers have relied on blind faith that their health has improved as a result of the pills they pop each morning. Quantitative measures of health may be able to shed light on whether that forty-dollar bottle is worth it each month. With personalized testing, we may no longer have to rely on the claims of others to determine what is best for our health and well-being.

As the science of biological aging measures continues to evolve, we will be able to learn more and more about ourselves. In my husband's case, I estimated a single biological age measure for him which, when compared to his chronological age, suggested he was on the right track. But as I mentioned in Part I of this book, aging is multidimensional. There isn't a single trajectory that we all move through, and some of us will be more prone to changing in one direction versus another. My lab has been able to quantitatively model this. By looking at thousands of variables measured in people's blood, we have been able to distinguish people with different aging trajectories. Some people will be more prone to accelerated metabolic changes, while others will experience a more pronounced rate of change in immune functioning.

As the science of aging continues to make progress, it also means that you may not have to go it alone. While one of the main goals of this book was to highlight the potential each of us has to impact our own aging process, I also feel it would be unjust to not mention the amazing progress that has been made when it comes to therapeutic aging interventions. My hope is that these will inspire you, rather than promote complacency. I have heard myself and many others say that some behavior that we do isn't a big deal because, by the time we are old, science will surely have a cure for that . . . Unfortunately, science can be painfully and disappointingly slow at times. Most of the scientists working on cancer during the mid-twentieth century would have never believed that we would still be without a cure today. Similarly, when President Bill Clinton announced the completion of sequencing the first draft of the human genome in 2000, it was predicted that it would revolutionize diagnosis and treatment of disease. As of now, we are still waiting for that dream to become reality.

Yet despite these setbacks, scientific progress over human history has been extraordinary. We captured electricity and put it into homes. We engineered flight. We walked on the moon. We built robotic personal assistants. While it may turn out that dramatically slowing our aging process and adding decades to healthspan and life span is too big a feat to tackle, the work being done by the thousands of teams of scientists across the world provides hope that a paradigm shift may be within our reach.

The current aging interventions on the horizon run the gamut from repurposing existing drugs to approaches once relegated to the realm of science fiction. While discussing all of them would require its own book, I would like to touch upon four that in my view represent some of the most promising avenues forward.

THE SECRETS BURIED IN THE SOIL

The first brings us back to the most successful aging intervention to date—CR, calorie restriction. I am not going to reiterate what I divulged in chapter 6 detailing the presumed benefits of restricting food intake. As mentioned, getting a large swath of the population to adopt such a protocol will be nearly impossible. That is not to say that we can't learn from CR, though, and discover the molecular remodeling that happens in response, then try to develop or identify pharmacological interventions that mimic it. These therapeutics are often referred to as "CR mimetics" and the goal is to give someone the benefits bestowed by CR through a pill rather than a lifestyle transformation.

In 2005, Dr. Matt Kaeberlein and others published a paper in *Science* demonstrating the impact of dietary restriction in yeast on the downregulation of a pathway called "TOR." Later it was shown that TOR (or mTOR in mammals) is an evolutionarily conserved network that, through cues from the environment, can alter basic cellular processes including growth (proliferation) and death (apoptosis). Basically, mTOR detects the levels of glucose/insulin, amino acids, leptin, and oxygen within cells, and when those are sufficiently high it will turn on, signaling to the body that it is time to grow. Conversely, when these inputs are low (as in the case of CR), mTOR will turn off, suggesting to the body that it should wait for more optimal conditions before ramping up growth. Because mTOR is thought to be responsible for many of the metabolic and immune shifts that occur in response to restricted food intake, it was hypothesized that manipulating this pathway could trick the body into thinking that it was undergoing CR, even when it wasn't.

Further evidence for the potential antiaging effects of blocking mTOR came in the form of genetic studies in which a number of labs showed that knocking out genes in the pathway could dramatically increase the life span of various organisms. This mounting evidence was a convincing first step to suggest that mTOR activation may have an evolutionarily ingrained function of regulating aging. Yet perhaps the most exciting thing was that a drug that could turn down mTOR activity had already been discovered forty years prior.

In November 1964, a team of physicians and scientists embarked on a journey from Halifax, Nova Scotia, to a tiny volcanic Polynesian island in the South Pacific known natively as Rapa Nui, but often referred to by others as Easter Island. This region had long held fascination as an archaeological site, as it is home to approximately nine hundred monolithic humanoid statues, called *mo'ai*, each standing about thirteen feet tall on average and weighing in at just under fourteen tons. On this expedition, however, the visitors were not there to investigate the five- to eight-hundred-year-old statues, but instead were intent on studying the health and environment of the current human inhabitants of the remote island.

As part of this project, one goal was to divide the island into parcels from which to collect soil samples. The goal was to understand how the residents of Easter Island avoided bacterial infection despite cohabitating with large numbers of livestock. While not much was gleaned from the initial screening of the vials of soil, twenty-five years later, while searching for bacterial-derived medicinal compounds, scientists at Ayerst Pharmaceuticals (today called Wyeth Pharmaceuticals) discovered something miraculous within the dirt: a bacteria with an ability to produce a power molecule that was subsequently named "rapamycin."

Over time, it was discovered that rapamycin was an extraordinary immunosuppressant, which is why one of its first applications was in organ transplants to prevent tissue rejection. It was also discovered that rapamycin could slow cellular growth, positioning it as a promising contender in the fight against cancer. Finally, in 2009, scientists observed that administration of rapamycin increased survival in male and female mice by 9 and 14 percent, respectively. What's more, it didn't seem to matter how old the mice were when treatment started.

Similar effects were shown for mice starting the regimen early in life (equivalent to a thirty-year-old human) or late in life (equivalent to a sixty-five-year-old human), providing the first proof of principle that pharmacological interventions could impact life span even when administered in late life.

Following the publication of these results, a plethora of closely related molecules, called "rapalogs," have been developed, and a number of clinical trials have been launched looking at their effects across an array of aging outcomes and various species. For instance, in mice, rapamycin has since been linked to decreases in heart disease, cancer, and brain aging. More recently, Dr. Kaeberlein and a fellow professor, Dr. Daniel Promislow, at the University of Washington, launched a trial through their Dog Aging Project, which is a large-scale study that seeks to investigate genetic and environmental mechanisms that regulate aging in domesticated dogs. Just like humans, dogs possess an enormous amount of genetic diversity, large variances in life span and disease risk, and often share environmental conditions with their human companions. As part of the larger project, the researchers sought to test whether rapamycin could improve cardiac health in healthy older dogs and determine optimal dosing. Based on promising results in the small pilot study, the team has hopes of scaling up and also examining other outcomes regarding cancer, kidney health, cognitive functioning, and various aging measures.

The multinational pharmaceutical company Novartis has also had its eye on rapalogs as a potential aging therapeutic. In 2014, they published their first human clinical trial results, showing that low-dose administration of one of their drugs boosted antibody response to the flu vaccine. Since then, Novartis's spin-off company, resTORbio—led by cofounder and chief medical officer Dr. Joan Mannick—has conducted a phase 3 trial for respiratory illness. Unfortunately, the trial failed to achieve their primary endpoints. While this may have slowed things down a bit, it in no way marks the end of rapalogs. Many researchers in the field of aging remain optimistic regarding the potential of rapalogs, and resTORbio is pushing forward with other clinical trials for aging-related diseases.

Yet even if rapalogs eventually prove successful at impacting aging in humans, that doesn't mean we should all jump on the bandwagon. Overall, scientists feel fairly confident when it comes to their efficacy, but less is known about potential side effects when it comes to long-term use. The FDA has approved rapamycin and rapalogs for transplants and pancreatic cancer therapy, but in both these cases, the anticipated benefits outweigh the potential side effects. But when it comes to administration in healthy individuals, that cost-benefit analysis is a bit less clear. Regardless, there are a number of aging-related diseases for which the use of rapamycin or rapalogs to treat them should be strongly considered.

KILLING ZOMBIES

Alzheimer's disease currently has no known treatments or cures. Diagnosis is a death sentence that carries with it the prospect of years of potential suffering for both the afflicted and their families. Remarkably, rapamycin has been shown to prevent cognitive decline and accumulating Alzheimer's disease pathology across ten studies using seven different mouse models of the disease. One potential mechanism through which this may occur is via rapamycin's ability to block and/or reduce the burden of senescent cells. Recall that senescent cells are often old or damaged cells that are resistant to cell death and instead stick around and chronically excrete pro-inflammatory factors that end up damaging neighboring cells and tissues. This toxic expression phenotype, referred

to as SASP (senescence-associated secretory phenotype), has been implicated in the progression of a number of diseases, including, recently,
Alzheimer's disease.

This brings us to our second potentially promising therapeutic, senolytics. Senolytics are a class of drugs that target senescent cells by forcing
them to commit cellular suicide (apoptosis). Once the cells are dead, they
can be cleared out and recycled. The last decade has spurred enormous
interest in the role of senescent cells in aging. They have been shown to
be major contributors of the accelerated aging phenotypes in models of
progeria syndromes and are linked to a wide array of diseases of aging.
But it took scientists showing that removal of these cells could ameliorate
signs of aging for biotech and pharmaceutical companies to start taking
note—and in a big way.

In 2011, a team of eight scientists at the Mayo Clinic that consisted
of Darren Baker, Tobias Wijshake, Tamar Tchkonia, Nathan LeBras-
seur, Bennett Childs, Bart van de Sluis, James Kirkland, and Jan van
Deursen designed a mouse model that could selectively target cells
harboring a marker of senescence called "p16INK4a." When a drug-
inducing death in these cells was administered, they found that the mice
went on to exhibit signs of postponement or even regression for a variety
of age-related phenotypes. This was even true for progeria mice who
would age at an accelerated rate naturally. This groundbreaking study
published in *Nature* provided the first proof of principle that senescence
may drive biological aging, and thus eliminating these cells could improve tissue functioning and prolong healthspan. There was a catch,
however. The model was done with what is called a "transgenic mouse,"
meaning that it was genetically modified. To do this in humans would
require the discovery of drugs that could act without the genetic ma-
nipulation.

Following the publication of the paper, van Deursen teamed up with
biotech entrepreneur Nathaniel "Ned" David, Dr. Daohong Zhou of the
University of Arkansas for Medical Sciences, and famed senescence

researcher Dr. Judy Campisi, a professor at the Buck Institute for Research on Aging in the San Francisco Bay Area. Campisi had been working on a transgenic mouse model similar to what was shown in van Deursen's paper. Together, they created the biotech start-up Unity, aimed at developing senolytic drugs that could eventually be used in humans.

Simultaneously, Dr. James Kirkland, one of the other authors on the original paper, was also on the hunt for drugs to target and kill senescent cells. In fact, Kirkland had already been working on this puzzle for more than half a decade. With his team at Mayo and scientists like Dr. Laura Niedernhofer (formerly at Scripps Research Institute and now at the University of Minnesota), Kirkland set out to identify pathways that are specific to senescent cells. The idea is that such targets would enable the team to selectively kill senescent cells while sparing the neighboring normal cells.

The problem is that, while we label a certain cellular phenotype as being senescent, the truth is these cells are very diverse. There is no single feature that has been discovered that distinguishes senescent from non-senescent cells. Because of this, initial targeting paradigms were not successful. Kirkland's team, however, knew that senescent cells as a whole all shared the characteristic of being impervious to the signals that tell a cell to undergo suicide. Thus, they hypothesized that disrupting this pathway could trigger senescent cells to undergo cell death. Eventually, through the help of bioinformatics, they discovered several potential pathways that seemed to underlie this adaptation of senescent cells. Interestingly, some of these pathways are also used by cancer cells to avoid death.

They also discovered two existing drugs that appeared effective in targeting these pathways. The drugs did not appear to work universally, though. One was effective for killing certain types of senescent cells, like those found in adipose tissues, while the other was effective against cells like those lining blood vessels. By simultaneously administering the two compounds to mice, the group demonstrated that they could produce the one-two punch needed for ameliorating some severe diseases of aging, including models of Alzheimer's disease and a chronic lung disease called "idiopathic pulmonary fibrosis" (IPF). The good news was, one of the drugs, dasatinib, was already FDA-approved, while the other, quercetin, was a plant-derived supplement.

Unity was also making headway in their drug discovery pipeline and, within a few years, had two promising candidates that had arisen from research in both the Campisi and Zhou labs. Today there are more than a dozen large public and private companies developing senolytics, and a growing number of other smaller start-ups with the potential to become real contenders. Unity completed a clinical trial on osteoarthritis for its leading drug candidate in 2020 but was unfortunately met with disappointing results. That only moderately disrupted the scientific enthusiasm in targeting senescence as a means to slow biological aging. Even if one candidate doesn't work (or at least not perfectly), that doesn't mean the concept is flawed. The evidence surrounding the ability of accumulating senescent cells to drive aging continues to mount every day. Aside from showing that eliminating them could slow aging, Kirkland has shown that injecting senescent cells into mice produced the reverse effect—an acceleration of aging phenotypes. There is also evidence surfacing that pairing senolytics with toxic treatments like chemotherapy and/or radiation could ameliorate adverse outcomes and the likelihood of cancer remission.

As we move forward down the path to developing more effective senolytics, it is important to keep in mind that senescent cells are not inherently bad. They exist for a reason, namely senescence is a detour for cells that are on the path to becoming cancerous. The toxic environment produced as more and more of our cells become senescent over time can drive biological aging; therefore, an alternative to directly targeting senescent cells per se is to target and remove the products of senescent cells (SASPs).

YOUNG BLOOD

One way to do this may be by diluting the problematic factors circulating around our bodies and cleaning up the environment our cells live in. You can think of this much in the same way we might think about our global environment, which, over time, has become more toxic. Over human history, the Earth's atmosphere has seen a rise in greenhouse gas emissions, air pollution, and smog, and infusion of inorganics like microplastics into our environment. As these factors accumulate, they can inflict damage on living organisms. A similar thing is thought to be happening inside our bodies—although in this context the accumulating factors likely include things like SASPs and inflammatory factors, oxidized products, and cross-linked or aggregated proteins, among others. Over time, these factors may impact cell functioning and lead to the age-related decline we observe in our various tissues and organs.

But what would happen if we could restore the environment back to what it once was? On Earth, we would imagine that this might restore the natural balance of our ecosystem. The same may be true in our bodies, as evidenced by some seemingly unorthodox experiments dating back hundreds of years.

In the mid-nineteenth century, French physiologist Paul Bert began a series of experiments in which he showed that it was possible to surgically connect the circulatory systems of two white albino rats, resulting in a single shared system. By the 1950s and 1960s, this technique, later termed "parabiosis" from the Greek *para* (alongside) and *bios* (life), started to be used to test the impact of blood composition on an animal's life span. These early studies provided the first hint that sharing a circulatory system with a younger animal could (for all intents and purposes) "rejuvenate" an old animal. While small, the studies showed that the pairing of an old animal with a young animal could improve metabolism and increase life span. Over the decades that followed, research into parabiosis fell by the wayside, and it wasn't until its reemergence starting in the early twenty-first century that researchers began to uncover how circulating factors in our blood both drive or turn back the aging clock.

In a Stanford lab in the early 2000s, a team of scientists that consisted of Irina and Michael Conboy, Amy Wagers, Eric Girma, Irving Weissman, and Thomas Rando began testing the impact of the circulating environment on skeletal muscle and hepatic (liver) stem cells. Typically, aging is accompanied by functional declines in these stem cells, leading to less regenerative capacity, an overall decline in muscle size/ strength, and impairments in metabolism and detoxification. The team observed that when old animals were connected to young ones so that they shared the same circulatory system, however, these age-related changes were attenuated. Subsequent studies by the same group and others have further affirmed that exposure to young blood can rejuvenate many of the aging-related changes that we once considered irreversible— including, it seems, brain aging. Research has also demonstrated that animals don't need to be connected to reap the benefits, and that simply exchanging things like blood plasma and serum can elicit similar responses. Interestingly, it has also since been shown that exposure to old blood prematurely ages a young animal, suggesting that it works in both directions.

Thus, the next logical step for the scientific community was to discover what was in the blood of old versus young animals that seemed to have such a profound effect on cellular aging. Just based on the parabiosis experiments, it wasn't clear whether the benefit to an old animal was due to a dilution of the problematic factors in their blood, or rather to the rejuvenating capacity of youthful factors contained in young blood. What's more, this is a critical component when it comes to developing feasible intervention strategies based on this work. While some companies prematurely jumped on the bandwagon and started offering "young [cell-free] blood" as an antiaging serum, most scientists and biotech start-ups in this realm were interested in a less vampire-esque route. The vast majority agreed that by discovering the secrets of *why* parabiosis had the power to accelerate or decelerate aging, we could focus on more targeted and safer ways to deliver the same benefit artificially. What's more, this approach wouldn't require droves of our young citizens lining up to provide samples from which to produce magical elixirs to restore youth and vitality for their elders.

So far, we haven't discovered the magic ingredients in young blood, although a number of labs and companies are investing heavily in this quest. What's more, a recent study from the Conboy Lab suggests that there isn't anything special about our blood when we are young, and that simply diluting old blood with a mixture of saline and albumin can achieve similar results. If so, this suggests that the factors floating around in our circulation may be in part what is driving our bodies to age. In the end, it may be that both are at play. Decreasing the concentration of the bad stuff will clearly be beneficial, but there are also things that may promote a healthier and more youthful environment.

Take, for instance, the research by Dr. Saul Villeda at UCSF that I discussed in chapter 8. His lab showed that when the blood of exercised mice was administered to non-exercised mice, they saw appreciable effects in terms of cognition and presumably slower brain aging. They were also able to isolate a protein that they suggested was responsible. Related work on exercise mimetics is also ongoing in the lab of Dr. Constanza (Connie) Cortes Rodriguez at the University of Alabama at Birmingham. Her lab has been able to design a mouse model that activates a gene that is typically induced after exercise. In a sense, they have tricked the muscles of the mouse into thinking that they just completed an aerobics class. While the research is still ongoing, the Cortes lab has observed remarkable remodeling in various other organs, from liver to pancreas, and even the brains of Alzheimer's mice. Suffice to say that the links among factors in our bodies and functioning of our cells is complicated. There are clearly some things that will accelerate our decline, while others may be able to restore youthful qualities.

REPROGRAMMING OUR OPERATING SYSTEM

Nowhere is this last point better illustrated than in the cutting-edge research involving what we call "cellular" or "epigenetic reprogramming." As I mentioned previously, every cell in a body shares essentially the same fixed genome. Yes, mutations arise, but in essence, our genome is set. This raises the questions: How do cells with the exact same genes take on so many diverse phenotypes? What determines if a cell is an embryonic stem cell or an adult neural brain cell? The answer is, our epigenome. Within each cell, the epigenome is a master conductor that directs information coded within the DNA of each cell to produce unique phenotypes. Overall, differences in the epigenetic pattern between cells is what generates the diversity within our tissues. The epigenome controls the rate at which new cells are made, determines the physical structure/shape of cells, dictates cellular responses to stress, and helps maintain stability of cell populations. Unfortunately, as with most things, this amazing biological operating system acquires glitches and becomes misconstrued over time, wreaking havoc on our bodies and potentially driving development of diseases of aging. But what if, much like our trusty AppleCare experts might restore the operating system of a failing MacBook, scientists could uncover a way to reprogram the declining epigenetic system? It might sound like a radical notion. After all, we are not computers and biology must be much more complex than IT. Well, maybe not . . .

In 2006, a groundbreaking discovery revolutionized how we think about epigenetics, cell identity, and even aging. Dr. Shinya Yamanaka, a professor of stem cell biology at the Institute for Frontier Medical Sciences at Kyoto University, Japan, wanted to discover the factors that determine a cell's identity. Working with his then postdoc assistant Dr. Kazutoshi Takahashi, the two took on the seemingly enormous challenge of trying to convert adult cells back into embryonic stem cells. They started by looking at the genes that were expressed by embryonic stem cells with the idea that some may be bestowing the unique characteristics of these cells, like the ability to develop into any number of cell types. They identified twenty-four potential protein factors that they believed might control the program of an embryonic stem cell. When all the factors were administered to the skin cells of an adult mouse, they observed something truly remarkable: the cells transformed into cells resembling embryonic stem cells. Through a series of other experiments, they were able to show that no factor could do this when administered on its own, but that a combination of just four factors (OCT 3/4, SOX2, KLF4, and MYC—OSKM for short) could do the trick. These genes would come to be known as "Yamanaka factors," studied by scientists worldwide, and go on to earn Shinya Yamanaka the Nobel Prize in medicine in 2012.

The potential of Yamanaka factors spans the gamut in science and medicine. In labs, they are being used to generate different cell types, like human neurons, so that they can be studied in dishes to better understand disease without needing to harvest cells from donated postmortem brains. For instance, biologists are able to take a skin sample from a person with Alzheimer's disease and a person free from disease, convert these both to stem cells (referred to as "induced pluripotent stem cells," or iPSCs), and then push the stem cells to develop into neurons that can be looked at to understand differences between neurons from people with neurodegenerative disease versus those without. In medicine, iPSCs are transforming regenerative therapies. Rather than needing to rely on embryonic stem cells, which carry a heavy moral and regulatory burden, doctors are now able to generate stem cells from their patients' own skin. So how does this fit with aging? To me, one of the most remarkable things about this discovery is the finding that reprogramming with Yamanaka factors also appears to rest our cells' aging clock.

If I were to take a skin sample of a fifty-year-old man and estimate biological age based on DNA methylation (epigenetics), chances are the resulting age estimate would be somewhere between forty-five and fifty years old. If I were to take that same sample and express Yamanaka factors and then reassess epigenetic age two weeks later, the sample would now have an epigenetic age of less than *zero*, suggesting that it is from a prenatal individual! This suggests that the aging pattern and the changes that we always assumed were just random accumulation of damage are reprogrammable. Our cells can be converted back to younger versions of themselves, and this youthful default state is in all of us. All we have to do is flip the switch.

In recent years, we have found that this switch from old to young cells not only occurs for cells in a dish but can also be initiated for cells in a body. In 2020, Dr. Yuancheng Lu, who was a graduate student in Dr. David Sinclair's lab at Harvard at the time, used Yamanaka factors to reprogram the cells in the optical nerves of mice. In doing so, the team was able to restore damage-induced or glaucoma-related vision loss, and in collaboration with my lab, we showed that they were also able to reverse the epigenetic age of these cells.

Other labs have also provided early evidence of the amazing potential of reprogramming biological aging. Dr. Juan Carlos Izpisua Belmonte of the Salk Institute in La Jolla, California, used reprogramming to delay or even reverse aging in mice. In the study, his team tested whether resetting the epigenome was enough to offset mutations that caused accelerated aging in progeria mice. They did not do anything to alter the mutations themselves, but showed that restoring a more youthful epigenome could extend the life spans of the mice by eighteen to twenty-four weeks (equivalent to around eight years for a human). When looking at "normal" mice, they also found that reprogramming could counter a number of age-related manifestations, including boosting resistance to metabolic disease and muscle loss.

Yet, besides providing a proof of concept for targeting aging via epigenetic reprogramming, the study also highlighted a critical point. Unlike the reprogramming studies of cells in culture, Izpisua Belmonte and his team undertook a protocol that they called "partial" or "cyclic" reprogramming, which meant that Yamanaka factors were only turned on for a short time (two days rather than weeks). The reason for this was because long-term expression of Yamanaka factors had been shown to be lethal and induced the formation of cancers, called "teratomas." Teratomas are rare tumors that comprise a variety of different developed tissues and organs, oftentimes things like teeth, hair, bone, and muscles. The reason this was happening in reprogrammed mice was because the fully developed cells that made up the different organs in the mouse's body were being converted back to stemlike cells that could then become other types of cells. Livers were no longer made of majority liver cells but rather stem cells, and a resulting hodgepodge of other cell types arose. Obviously, this is not what we want.

Luckily, what Izpisua Belmonte and others have discovered is that during the process of reprogramming, the aging signature is the first thing to be reversed, before the cells convert back to stemlike states. Thus, Izpisua Belmonte showed that by turning off the treatment *before* the cells converted (or what is called "dedifferentiated"), they could reverse aging while retaining the cells' original identity. Epigenetic aging patterns were rejuvenated and now what was once an old liver cell is just a younger liver cell.

There are still a number of questions that need to be answered before epigenetic reprogramming can be considered a viable treatment in humans. For instance, we don't know how long the treatment should be applied. It may be cell and/or tissue specific. We don't know if there are better combinations of reprogramming factors or mechanisms that can prevent the dedifferentiation of cells. We don't know how long this effect would last. Remember from the parabiosis experiments that young cells exposed to (or inside of) an old environment will age faster. We also don't know whether we can do this for an entire body or if there are specific organs and cells that should be targeted to elicit the greatest benefit. We also don't know how many times we can safely do this and still see appreciable benefits with limited risk.

Even on a more basic level, we have yet to determine how nature and biology accomplish this amazing feat. Somehow it seems that cells have memory. They are able to return to an epigenetic state that closely resembles the past and, for all intents and purposes, it is hard to distinguish between a true embryonic stem cell and an old cell that has simply been converted. Despite all these unanswered questions, this amazing phenomenon confirms that aging is malleable. While time's arrow may point in one direction, biology doesn't have to.

WHY WAIT?

Strategies like epigenetic reprogramming may help future humans turn back the clock and escape many of the diseases of aging. Conversely, it also may be the case that this strategy does not pan out, despite the best efforts and hours of dedication from brilliant scientists around the globe. Humans are constantly striving to push the boundaries of what is possible in science and technology, to improve ourselves beyond what we thought was possible. When it comes to optimizing health and aging, betterment doesn't have to come via a pill bottle or through the needle's tip at the end of a syringe. While we wait for those groundbreaking discoveries, there are things each of us can do for ourselves.

By understanding and tracking our own aging process, we can discover ways to delay our own aging, discover habits that work for us, determine whether to seek medical advice before we are ever sick, and be accountable for our own health and wellness as we enjoy our chronological time on Earth.

CONFLICTS OF INTEREST

As a closing, I want to formally acknowledge some of my financial ties that could be seen as potential conflicts of interest in relation to what I covered in this book. It was never my intention to use this platform as a means to sell or promote the products that I have helped develop. Through this book, it was always my goal to educate readers on the various options and ways one might track the aging process. It is true that in doing so, I have mentioned products and/or companies that I have links to. Some of the tools I have developed, however, are also freely available. Through my work and my personal health endeavors, I have come to recognize the enormous potential of biological age tracking and, as such, feel strongly that it should be a possibility for everyone. I sincerely believe that science and technology should not serve as a means to further propagate the health disparities that plague modern societies. Instead, science should be seen as a tool for closing those gaps. When it comes down to it, a nation is only as healthy as its least healthy citizens.

NOTES

1. BEYOND WRINKLES: THE LINK BETWEEN HEALTH AND AGING

12 **First performed in 1889:** A. Ghossain and M. A. Ghossain, "History of Mastectomy Before and After Halsted," *Lebanese Medical Journal* 52, no. 2 (2009): 65–71.

14 **8 out of 10 COVID-19 deaths:** CDC, *COVID-19*, "Older Adults: At Greater Risk of Requiring Hospitalization or Dying if Diagnosed with COVID-19," https://www.cdc.gov/coronavirus/2019-ncov/need-extra-precautions/older-adults.html.

15 **"older people die":** C. K. Chumley, "Coronavirus Case and Death Counts in U.S. Ridiculously Low," *Washington Times*, April 14, 2020.

16 **mortality risk from nearly every major disease:** S. J. Olshansky, "Articulating the Case for the Longevity Dividend," *Cold Spring Harbor Perspectives in Medicine* 6, no. 2 (February 2016): a025940.

2. WHY TO TRACK YOUR TRUE AGE

22 **Tobacco smoke comprises over 7,000 chemicals:** CDC, *How Tobacco Smoke Causes Disease: The Biology and Behavioral Basis for Smoking-Attributable Disease: A Report of the Surgeon General*, Centers for Disease Control and Prevention, 2012.

32 **five-day fasting-mimicking diet:** M. Wei et al., "Fasting-Mimicking Diet and Markers/Risk Factors for Aging, Diabetes, Cancer, and Cardiovascular Disease," *Science Translational Medicine* 9, no. 377 (February 2017): https://doi:10.1126/scitranslmed.aai8700.

3. WHAT IS BIOLOGICAL AGING?

41 **are identical to that of a mouse:** W. Makalowski, J. Zhang, and M. S. Boguski, "Comparative Analysis of 1196 Orthologous Mouse and Human Full-Length mRNA and Protein Sequences," *Genome Research* 6, no. 9 (September 1996): 846–57.

42 **lens crystallins in the eyes of Greenland sharks:** J. Nielsen et al., "Eye Lens Radio-Carbon Reveals Centuries of Longevity in the Greenland Shark (*Somniosus microcephalus*)," *Science* 353, no. 6300 (August 2016): 702–4.

42 **Within the honeybee colony:** E. O. Wilson, *The Insect Societies* (Cambridge, MA: Belknap Press, 1971), x, 548.

42 drones have half as many chromosomes: G. M. Weinstock et al., "Insights into Social Insects from the Genome of the Honeybee *Apis mellifera*," *Nature* 443, no. 7114 (October 2006): 931–49.

43 The larva queen feasts on "royal jelly": M. H. Haydak, "Honey Bee Nutrition," *Annual Review of Entomology* 15, no. 143 (January 1970): 143–56.

48 altered epigenetic patterns: W. Zhou et al., "DNA Methylation Loss in Late-Replicating Domains Is Linked to Mitotic Cell Division," *Nature Genetics* 50, no. 4 (April 2018): 591–602.

48 we can observe the same epigenetic changes: C. Minteer et al., "A DNAmRep Epigenetic Fingerprint for Determining Cellular Replication Age," *bioRxiv* (2020): https://doi.org/10.1101/2020.09.02.280073.

49 Discovered by Dr. Barbara McClintock in the 1950s: B. McClintock, "The Origin and Behavior of Mutable Loci in Maize," *PNAS* 36, no. 6 (June 1950): 344–55.

50 a German biologist by the name of August Weismann: A. Weismann, *Essays upon Heredity and Kindred Biological Problems*, 2nd ed. (Oxford, UK: Clarendon Press, 1891).

50 Hayflick and Moorhead showed that cells: L. Hayflick and P. S. Moorhead, "The Serial Cultivation of Human Diploid Cell Strains," *Experimental Cell Research* 25, no. 3 (December 1961): 585–621.

51 discovered the protein telomerase: C. W. Greider and E. H. Blackburn, "Identification of a Specific Telomere Terminal Transferase Activity in Tetrahymena Extracts," *Cell* 43, no. 2, pt. 1 (December 1985): 405–13.

52 Cellular senescence is a stress-induced state: J. P. de Magalhães and J. F. Passos, "Stress, Cell Senescence and Organismal Ageing," *Mechanisms of Ageing and Development* 170 (March 2018): 2–9.

52 senescent cells chronically activate pro-inflammatory genes: J. -P. Coppé et al., "The Senescence-Associated Secretory Phenotype: The Dark Side of Tumor Suppression," *Annual Review of Pathology* 5 (2010): 99–118.

53 the supply of adult stem cells is not endless: J. Oh, Y. D. Lee, and A. J. Wagers, "Stem Cell Aging: Mechanisms, Regulators and Therapeutic Opportunities," *Nature Medicine* 20, no. 8 (August 2014): 870–80.

53 detectable white blood cell mutation: S. Jaiswal et al., "Age-Related Clonal Hematopoiesis Associated with Adverse Outcomes," *New England Journal of Medicine* 371, no. 26 (December 2014): 2488–98.

54 a paper by the brilliant British physician and biologist Dr. John Cairns: J. Cairns, "Mutation Selection and the Natural History of Cancer," *Nature* 255, no. 5505 (May 1975): 197–200.

55 directs the actions of the subsequent cells: D. Lehotzky and G. K. H. Zupanc, "Cellular Automata Modeling of Stem-Cell-Driven Development of Tissue in the Nervous System," *Developmental Neurobiology* 79, no. 5 (May 2019): 497–517.

56 Each one of us is strongly influenced by the inputs: N. A. Christakis, "Social Networks and Collateral Health Effects," *BMJ* 329, no. 7459 (July 2004): 184–85.

56 These include overpopulation: A. Brooks, "Guns, Germs and Steel: A Short History of Everybody for the Last 13,000 Years," *BMJ* 318, no. 7193 (May 1999): 1294A.

57 cells that once had specific identities: J.-H. Yang et al., "Erosion of the Epigenetic Landscape and Loss of Cellular Identity as a Cause of Aging in Mammals," *bioRxiv* (October 2019): https://doi.org/10.1101/808642.

58 the "adaptive oncogenesis model": A. Marusyk and J. DeGregori, "Declining Cellular Fitness with Age Promotes Cancer Initiation by Selecting for Adaptive Oncogenic Mutations," *Biochimica et Biophysica Acta* 1785, no. 1 (January 2008): 1–11.

61 Alzheimer's disease is a progressive degeneration: Alzheimer's Association, "What Is Alzheimer's Disease?," accessed 2021, https://www.alz.org/alzheimers-dementia/what-is-alzheimers.

62 senescent cells may be prevalent in Alzheimer's: P. Zhang et al., "Senolytic Therapy Alleviates Aβ-Associated Oligodendrocyte Progenitor Cell Senescence and Cognitive Deficits in an Alzheimer's Disease Model," *Nature Neuroscience* 22, no. 5 (May 2019): 719–28.

4. HOW TO MEASURE BIOLOGICAL AGE

67 known as "the Frailty Index": K. Rockwood and A. Mitnitski, "Frailty in Relation to the Accumulation of Deficits," *Journals of Gerontology*, series A, *Biological Sciences and Medical Sciences* 62, no. 7 (July 2007): 722–27.

70 One method, called "qPCR": J. Lin et al., "Telomere Length Measurement by qPCR—Summary of Critical Factors and Recommendations for Assay Design," *Psychoneuroendocrinology* 99 (January 2019): 271–78.

70 psychological stress was associated with shorter telomere length: E. S. Epel et al., "Accelerated Telomere Shortening in Response to Life Stress," *PNAS* 101, no. 49 (December 2004): 17312.

73 aging measure that combined multidimensional information: M. E. Levine et al., "An Epigenetic Biomarker of Aging for Lifespan and Healthspan," *Aging* (Albany, NY) 10, no. 4 (April 2018): 573–91.

75 estimated the relative influence: Z. Liu et al., "Associations of Genetics, Behaviors, and Life Course Circumstances with a Novel Aging and Healthspan Measure: Evidence from the Health and Retirement Study," *PLoS Medicine* 16, no. 6 (June 2019): e1002827.

76 highlighting the astounding financial investment: V. Moorhouse, "How Much We Spend on Anti-Aging Cream over a Lifetime Is ASTOUNDING," *InStyle*, October 12, 2018.

77 John Carreyrou in his book, *Bad Blood*: J. Carreyrou, *Bad Blood: Secrets and Lies in a Silicon Valley Startup* (New York: Knopf, 2018).

78 DNA methylation patterns that seemed to distinguish cancerous tissues: N. Ahuja et al., "Aging and DNA Methylation in Colorectal Mucosa and Cancer," *Cancer Research* 58, no. 23 (December 1998): 5489–94.

79 an "epigenetic clock": S. Bocklandt et al., "Epigenetic Predictor of Age," *PLoS ONE* 6, no. 6 (June 2011): e14821.

79 **the second DNA methylation age predictor:** G. Hannum et al., "Genome-Wide Methylation Profiles Reveal Quantitative Views of Human Aging Rates," *Molecular Cell* 49, no. 2 (January 2013): 359–67.

80 **Dr. Horvath developed:** S. Horvath, "DNA Methylation Age of Human Tissues and Cell Types," *Genome Biology* 14, no. 3156 (December 2013).

80 **menopause tended to accelerate epigenetic aging:** M. E. Levine et al., "Menopause Accelerates Biological Aging," *PNAS* 113, no. 33 (July 2016): 9327–32.

80 **predictive of future risk of lung cancer:** M. E. Levine et al., "DNA Methylation Age of Blood Predicts Future Onset of Lung Cancer in the Women's Health Initiative," *Aging* (Albany, NY) 7, no. 9 (September 2015): 690–700.

81 **people who ate more leafy greens:** A. Quach et al., "Epigenetic Clock Analysis of Diet, Exercise, Education, and Lifestyle Factors," *Aging* (Albany, NY) 9, no. 2 (February 2017): 419–37.

81 **insomnia was linked to faster epigenetic aging:** J. E. Carroll et al., "Epigenetic Aging and Immune Senescence in Women with Insomnia Symptoms: Findings from the Women's Health Initiative Study," *Biological Psychiatry* 18, no. 2 (January 2017): 136–44.

81 **difference between epigenetic age and chronological age:** B. H. Chen et al., "DNA Methylation-Based Measures of Biological Age: Meta-Analysis Predicting Time to Death," *Aging* (Albany, NY) 8, no. 9 (September 2016): 1844–65.

83 **better predictor for myriad health outcomes:** Levine et al., "An Epigenetic Biomarker of Aging for Lifespan and Healthspan."

84 **a gene called "SIR2":** M. Kaeberlein, M. McVey, and L. Guarente, "The SIR2/3/4 Complex and SIR2 Alone Promote Longevity in *Saccharomyces cerevisiae* by Two Different Mechanisms," *Genes & Development* 13, no. 19 (October 1999): 2570–80.

85 **Without NAD, increasing the activation of SIR2:** S. Imai et al., "Transcriptional Silencing and Longevity Protein Sir2 Is an NAD-Dependent Histone Deacetylase," *Nature* 403, no. 6771 (February 2000): 795–800.

85 **family of proteins called "sirtuins":** S. Michan and D. Sinclair, "Sirtuins in Mammals: Insights into Their Biological Function," *Biochemical Journal* 404, no. 1 (May 2007): 1–13.

5. THE FUTURE OF PERSONALIZED AGING

92 **profiles they called "ageotypes":** S. Ahadi et al., "Personal Aging Markers and Ageotypes Revealed by Deep Longitudinal Profiling," *Nature Medicine* 26, no. 1 (January 2020): 83–90.

96 **median life expectancy at birth in 2018:** WorldData.info, "Life Expectancy for Men and Women," cited 2021, https://www.worlddata.info/life-expectancy.php.

96 **50 million people living with Alzheimer's disease:** M. K. Andrew and M. C. Tierney, "The Puzzle of Sex, Gender and Alzheimer's Disease: Why Are Women More Often Affected Than Men?," *Women's Health* 14 (December 2018): https://doi.org/10.1177/1745506518817995.

96 **81 percent of women over the age of ninety:** S. G. Leveille et al., "Sex Differences in the Prevalence of Mobility Disability in Old Age: The Dynamics of Incidence, Recovery, and Mortality," *Journals of Gerontology*, series B, *Psychological Sciences and Social Sciences* 56, no. 5 (September 2001): S294–301.

96 **"the male-female health survival paradox":** D. L. Wingard, "The Sex Differential in Morbidity, Mortality, and Lifestyle," *Annual Review of Public Health* 5 (1984): 433–58.

102 **an experiment led by Dr. Nan Hao:** Y. Li et al., "A Programmable Fate Decision Landscape Underlies Single-Cell Aging in Yeast," *Science* 369, no. 6501 (July 2020): 325–29.

105 **genetic profiles associated with accelerated aging:** C. -L. Kuo et al., "Genetic Associations for Two Biological Age Measures Point to Distinct Aging Phenotypes," *medRxiv* (July 2020): https://doi.org/10.1101/2020.07.10.20150797.

6. EAT (LESS) TO LIVE

127 **"Those that feed":** L. An, *The Huainanzi*, trans. and ed. John S. Major et al. (Columbia University Press, 2010): 161.

128 **reduction of caloric intake could slow:** C. Moreschi, "*Beziehungen Zwischen Ernährung und Tumorwachstum*," *Zeitschrift für Immunitätsforsch* 2 (1909): 651–75.

128 **a study by Dr. Peyton Rous:** P. Rous, "The Influence of Diet on Transplanted and Spontaneous Mouse Tumors," *Journal of Experimental Medicine* 20, no. 5 (November 1914): 433–51.

128 **his manuscript published in 1914:** Rous, "The Influence of Diet on Transplanted and Spontaneous Mouse Tumors," 450–51.

128 **rats whose growth had been nutritionally stunted:** T. B. Osborne, L. B. Mendel, and E. L. Ferry, "The Effect of Retardation of Growth upon the Breeding Period and Duration of Life of Rats," *Science* 45, no. 1160 (March 1917): 294–95.

129 **the discoverer of vitamins A and B:** L. Rosenfeld, "Vitamine—Vitamin: The Early Years of Discovery," *Clinical Chemistry* 43, no. 4 (1997): 680–85.

130 **demonstrate the longevity impact of CR:** C. M. McCay, M. F. Crowell, and L. A. Maynard, "The Effect of Retarded Growth upon the Length of Life Span and upon the Ultimate Body Size: One Figure," *Journal of Nutrition* 10, no. 1 (July 1935): 63–79.

133 **Biosphere 2 research facility:** Carl Zimmer, "The Lost History of One of the World's Strangest Science Experiments," *New York Times*, March 29, 2019.

134 **50 percent in rodents fed restricted diets:** R. Weindruch et al., "The Retardation of Aging in Mice by Dietary Restriction: Longevity, Cancer, Immunity and Lifetime Energy Intake," *Journal of Nutrition* 116, no. 4 (April 1986): 641–54.

138 **80 percent of their calorically restricted monkeys:** R. J. Colman et al., "Caloric Restriction Delays Disease Onset and Mortality in Rhesus Monkeys," *Science* 325, no. 5937 (July 2009): 201–4.

138 **"by following a special diet":** Nicholas Wade, "Dieting Monkeys Offer Hope for Living Longer," *New York Times*, July 9, 2009, https://www.nytimes.com/2009/07/10/science/10aging.html.

138 **the calorically restricted and the ad libitum–fed monkeys:** J. A. Mattison et al., "Impact of Caloric Restriction on Health and Survival in Rhesus Monkeys from the NIA Study," *Nature* 489, no. 7414 (September 2012): 318–21.

139 **similarities and differences between the two studies:** J. A. Mattison et al., "Caloric Restriction Improves Health and Survival of Rhesus Monkeys," *Nature Communications* 8, no. 14063 (January 2017): https://doi.org/10.1038/ncomms14063.

147 **people could be counted on to maintain a CR diet:** S. B. Racette et al., "One Year of Caloric Restriction in Humans: Feasibility and Effects on Body Composition and Abdominal Adipose Tissue," *Journals of Gerontology*, series A, *Biological Sciences and Medical Sciences* 61, no. 9 (September 2006): 943–50.

148 **simply maintain their current dietary practice:** E. Ravussin et al., "A 2-Year Randomized Controlled Trial of Human Caloric Restriction: Feasibility and Effects on Predictors of Health Span and Longevity," *Journals of Gerontology*, series A, *Biological Sciences and Medical Sciences* 70, no. 9 (July 2015): 1097–104.

148 **They were aging 87.5 percent slower:** D. W. Belsky et al., "Change in the Rate of Biological Aging in Response to Caloric Restriction: CALERIE Biobank Analysis," *Journals of Gerontology*, series A, *Biological Sciences and Medical Sciences* 73, no. 1 (December 2017): 4–10.

7. LONGEVITY DIETS

154 **the link between BMI and health outcomes:** Z. Liu et al., "A New Aging Measure Captures Morbidity and Mortality Risk Across Diverse Subpopulations from NHANES IV: A Cohort Study," *PLoS Medicine* 15, no. 12 (December 2018): e1002718.

156 **the number of fat cells in our bodies:** K. L. Spalding et al., "Dynamics of Fat Cell Turnover in Humans," *Nature* 453, no. 7196 (May 2008): 783–87.

158 **humans as "the fat primate":** D. Swain-Lenz et al., "Comparative Analyses of Chromatin Landscape in White Adipose Tissue Suggest Humans May Have Less Beigeing Potential Than Other Primates," *Genome Biology and Evolution* 11, no. 7 (July 2019): 1997–2008.

161 **plant-based or vegan diet and the Mediterranean diet:** M. A. Mendez and A. B. Newman, "Can a Mediterranean Diet Pattern Slow Aging?," *Journals of Gerontology*, series A 73, no. 3 (March 2018): 315–17.

162 **IGF-1 levels of humans on a CR diet:** L. Fontana et al., "Long-Term Effects of Calorie or Protein Restriction on Serum IGF-1 and IGFBP-3 Concentration in Humans," *Aging Cell* 7, no. 5 (October 2008): 681–87.

162 **low protein intake—particularly low animal protein:** M. E. Levine et al., "Low Protein Intake Is Associated with a Major Reduction in IGF-1, Cancer, and Overall Mortality in the 65 and Younger but Not Older Population," *Cell Metabolism* 19, no. 3 (March 2014): 407–17.

168 *most of their diet was derived from plants*: D. Buettner and S. Skemp, "Blue Zones: Lessons from the World's Longest Lived," *American Journal of Lifestyle Medicine* 10, no. 5 (September–October 2016): 318–21.

170 "belly 80 percent full": I. Rubaum-Keller, "Hara Hachi Bu: Eat Until You Are 80% Full," The Blog, *HuffPost*, September 21, 2011, https://www.huffpost.com/entry/not-overeating_b_969910.

171 Greek Orthodox practices of religious fasting: K. O. Sarri et al., "Effects of Greek Orthodox Christian Church Fasting on Serum Lipids and Obesity," *BMC Public Health* 3, no. 16 (May 2003), https://doi.org/10.1186/1471-2458-3-16.

172 Daoist text *Biographies of the Immortals*: M. LaFargue, review of *The Daoist Tradition: An Introduction*, by Louis Komjathy, *Religious Studies Review* 40, no. 2 (2014): 121.

172 put mice on an alternate-day fasting regimen: R. M. Anson et al., "Intermittent Fasting Dissociates Beneficial Effects of Dietary Restriction on Glucose Metabolism and Neuronal Resistance to Injury from Calorie Intake," *PNAS* 100, no. 10 (May 2003): 6216–20.

173 stumbled on the benefits of fasting: P. Jarreau, "5 Human Fasting Studies with Dr. Mark Mattson," LifeApps, March 14, 2019, https://lifeapps.io/fasting/5-human-fasting-studies-with-dr-mark-mattson/.

173 alternate-day fasting for three months: K. A. Varady et al., "Alternate Day Fasting for Weight Loss in Normal Weight and Overweight Subjects: A Randomized Controlled Trial," *Nutrition Journal* 12, no. 146 (November 2013): https://doi.org/10.1186/1475-2891-12-146.

180 A yearlong study of a hundred obese volunteers: J. F. Trepanowski et al., "Effect of Alternate-Day Fasting on Weight Loss, Weight Maintenance, and Cardioprotection Among Metabolically Healthy Obese Adults: A Randomized Clinical Trial," *JAMA Internal Medicine* 177, no. 7 (July 2017): 930–38.

182 subjects followed a ten-hour TRE protocol: M. J. Wilkinson et al., "Ten-Hour Time-Restricted Eating Reduces Weight, Blood Pressure, and Atherogenic Lipids in Patients with Metabolic Syndrome," *Cell Metabolism* 31, no. 1 (January 2020): 92–104.e5.

185 the keto diet may slow the rate of biological aging: M. N. Roberts et al., "A Ketogenic Diet Extends Longevity and Healthspan in Adult Mice," *Cell Metabolism* 26, no. 3 (September 2017): 539–46.e5.

186 drawbacks of long-term keto adoption: E. L. Goldberg et al., "Ketogenesis Activates Metabolically Protective γδ T Cells in Visceral Adipose Tissue," *Nature Metabolism* 2, no. 1 (January 2020): 50–61.

8. EXERCISE AND AGING

191 those who reported sitting the most: E. G. Wilmo et al., "Sedentary Time in Adults and the Association with Diabetes, Cardiovascular Disease and Death: Systematic Review and Meta-Analysis," *Diabetologia* 55, no. 11 (November 2012): 2895–905.

191 **shown to reverse type 2 diabetes:** S. R. Colberg et al., "Physical Activity/Exercise and Diabetes: A Position Statement of the American Diabetes Association," *Diabetes Care* 39, no. 11 (November 2016): 2065–79.

191 **activity has been linked to greater survival:** M. D. Holmes et al., "Physical Activity and Survival After Breast Cancer Diagnosis," *JAMA* 293, no. 20 (May 2005): 2479–86.

192 **thirteen different types of cancers:** S. C. Moore et al., "Association of Leisure-Time Physical Activity with Risk of 26 Types of Cancer in 1.44 Million Adults," *AMA Internal Medicine* 176, no. 6 (June 2016): 816–25.

192 **contributed to 5.3 million excess deaths:** I. -M. Lee et al., "Effect of Physical Inactivity on Major Non-Communicable Diseases Worldwide: An Analysis of Burden of Disease and Life Expectancy," *Lancet* 380, no. 9838 (July 2012): 219–29.

195 **boost the liver's ability to dispose of lactic acid:** G. A. Brooks, "The Science and Translation of Lactate Shuttle Theory," *Cell Metabolism* 27, no. 4 (April 2018): 757–85.

199 **an additive called "MF59 adjuvant":** K. Lindert et al., "Cumulative Clinical Experience with MF59-Adjuvanted Trivalent Seasonal Influenza Vaccine in Young Children and Adults 65 Years of Age and Older," *International Journal of Infectious Diseases* 85s (August 2019): S10–17.

200 **administered the blood from exercised mice:** A. M. Horowitz et al., "Blood Factors Transfer Beneficial Effects of Exercise on Neurogenesis and Cognition to the Aged Brain," *Science* 369, no. 6500 (July 2020): 167–73.

202 **Sarcopenia is also a major risk factor:** S. S. Y. Yeung et al., "Sarcopenia and Its Association with Falls and Fractures in Older Adults: A Systematic Review and Meta-Analysis," *Journal of Cachexia, Sarcopenia and Muscle* 10, no. 3 (June 2019): 485–500.

202 **increased muscle strength by 113 percent:** R. Bross, M. Javanbakht, and S. Bhasin, "Anabolic Interventions for Aging-Associated Sarcopenia," *Journal of Clinical Endocrinology & Metabolism* 84, no. 10 (October 1999): 3420–30.

205 **Mayo Clinic showed that three months of HIIT:** M. M. Robinson et al., "Enhanced Protein Translation Underlies Improved Metabolic and Physical Adaptations to Different Exercise Training Modes in Young and Old Humans," *Cell Metabolism* 25, no. 3 (March 2017): 581–92.

207 **U-shaped association between certain activities:** A. Merghani, A. Malhotra, and S. Sharma, "The U-Shaped Relationship Between Exercise and Cardiac Morbidity," *Trends in Cardiovascular Medicine* 26, no. 3 (April 2016): 232–40.

9. REST AND RELAXATION

216 **observe blood flow, CSF flow, and electrical activity:** N. E. Fultz et al., "Coupled Electrophysiological, Hemodynamic, and Cerebrospinal Fluid Oscillations in Human Sleep," *Science* 366, no. 6465 (November 2019): 628–31.

216 **in Alzheimer's, brains often accumulate two hallmarks:** A. Serrano-Pozo et al., "Neuropathological Alterations in Alzheimer Disease," *Cold Spring Harbor*

Perspectives in Medicine 1, no. 1 (September 2011); https://doi.org/10.1101/cshperspect.a006189.

220 **At the core of this timepiece are two genes:** E. D. Buhr and J. S. Takahashi, "Molecular Components of the Mammalian Circadian Clock," *Handbook of Experimental Pharmacology* 217 (September 2013): 3–27.

222 **SIRT1 activity in the brains of mice:** H. -C. Chang and L. Guarente, "SIRT1 Mediates Central Circadian Control in the SCN by a Mechanism That Decays with Aging," *Cell* 153, no. 7 (June 2013): 1448–60.

222 **a group of young adults was asked:** F. O. James, N. Cermakian, and D. B. Boivin, "Circadian Rhythms of Melatonin, Cortisol, and Clock Gene Expression During Simulated Night Shift Work," *Sleep* 30, no. 11 (November 2007): 1427–36.

225 **increases in rates of clinically significant insomnia:** C. M. Morin and J. Carrier, "The Acute Effects of the COVID-19 Pandemic on Insomnia and Psychological Symptoms," *Sleep Medicine* 77 (January 2021): 346–47.

226 **By tracking the profession status and health:** J. Caputo, E. K. Pavalko, and M. A. Hardy, "Midlife Work and Women's Long-Term Health and Mortality," *Demography* 57, no. 1 (December 2019): 373–402.

231 **A condition called Cushing's disease:** H. Ellis, "Harvey Cushing: Cushing's Disease," *Journal of Perioperative Practice* 22, no. 9 (September 2012): 298–99.

233 **"conserved transcriptional response to adversity," or CTRA:** S. W. Cole, "The Conserved Transcriptional Response to Adversity," *Current Opinion in Behavioral Sciences* 28 (August 2019): 31–37.

234 **embracing stress has the potential:** A. J. Crum, J. P. Jamieson, and M. Akinola, "Optimizing Stress: An Integrated Intervention for Regulating Stress Responses," *Emotion* 20, no. 1 (February 2020): 120–25.

235 **the most beneficial ways to think about stress:** Kelly McGonigal, *The Upside of Stress: Why Stress Is Good for You, and How to Get Good at It* (New York: Avery, 2015).

235 **those who engage in mindfulness training:** A. A. Taren et al., "Mindfulness Meditation Training Alters Stress-Related Amygdala Resting State Functional Connectivity: A Randomized Controlled Trial," *Social Cognitive and Affective Neuroscience* 10, no. 12 (June 2015): 1758–68.

238 **health disparities between the rich and the poor:** E. M. Crimmins, J. K. Kim, and T. E. Seeman, "Poverty and Biological Risk: The Earlier 'Aging' of the Poor," *Journals of Gerontology*, series A, *Biological Sciences and Medical Sciences* 64, no. 2 (February 2009): 286–92.

239 **what is deemed "worst-case housing needs":** N. E. Watson et al., *Worst Case Housing Needs: 2019 Report to Congress*, Washington, DC: U.S. Department of Housing and Urban Development, June 2020.

240 **most countries fall drastically short:** World Economic Forum, *Global Social Mobility Index 2020: Why Economies Benefit from Fixing Inequality*, January 2020.

240 **"the long arm of childhood":** M. D. Hayward and B. K. Gorman, "The Long Arm of Childhood: The Influence of Early-Life Social Conditions on Men's Mortality," *Demography* 41, no. 1 (February 2004): 87–107.

241 **the example of the Dutch Hunger Winter:** L. C. Schulz, "The Dutch Hunger Winter and the Developmental Origins of Health and Disease," *PNAS* 107, no. 39 (September 2010): 16757.

242 **epigenetic adaptations to food scarcity:** C. N. Hales and D. J. Barker, "The Thrifty Phenotype Hypothesis," *British Medical Bulletin* 60 (2001): 5–20.

243 **aging rates of individuals as a function of race:** M. E. Levine and E. M. Crimmins, "Evidence of Accelerated Aging Among African Americans and Its Implications for Mortality," *Social Science & Medicine* 118 (October 2014): 27–32.

243 **referred to as the "weathering hypothesis":** A. T. Geronimus, "The Weathering Hypothesis and the Health of African-American Women and Infants: Evidence and Speculations," *Ethnicity & Disease* 2, no. 3 (Summer 1992): 207–21.

10. FINDING YOUR "JUST RIGHT"

250 **23,000 emergency department visits:** A. I. Geller et al., "Emergency Department Visits for Adverse Events Related to Dietary Supplements," *New England Journal of Medicine* 373, no. 16 (October 2015): 1531–40.

252 **downregulation of a pathway called "TOR":** M. Kaeberlein et al., "Regulation of Yeast Replicative Life Span by TOR and Sch9 in Response to Nutrients," *Science* 310, no. 5751 (November 2005): 1193–96.

253 **In November 1964, a team of physicians and scientists:** Jacalyn Duffin, *Stanley's Dream: The Medical Expedition to Easter Island* (Montreal: McGill-Queen's University Press, 2019): 3.

253 **administration of rapamycin increased survival:** D. E. Harrison et al., "Rapamycin Fed Late in Life Extends Lifespan in Genetically Heterogeneous Mice," *Nature* 460, no. 7253 (July 2009): 392–95.

254 **boosted antibody response to the flu vaccine:** J. B. Mannick et al., "mTOR Inhibition Improves Immune Function in the Elderly," *Science Translational Medicine* 6, no. 268 (December 2014): 268ra179.

256 **a marker of senescence called "p16INK4a":** D. J. Baker et al., "Clearance of p16Ink4a-Positive Senescent Cells Delays Ageing-Associated Disorders," *Nature* 479, no. 7372 (November 2011): 232–36.

257 **underlie this adaptation of senescent cells:** Y. Zhu et al., "The Achilles' Heel of Senescent Cells: From Transcriptome to Senolytic Drugs," *Aging Cell* 14, no. 4 (August 2015): 644–58.

259 **surgically connect the circulatory systems:** P. Bert, "Sur la Greffe Animale," *Comptes rendus de l'académie des sciences* 61 (1865): 587–89.

260 **impact of the circulating environment:** I. M. Conboy et al., "Rejuvenation of Aged Progenitor Cells by Exposure to a Young Systemic Environment," *Nature* 433, no. 7027 (February 2005): 760–64.

261 **diluting old blood with a mixture of saline and albumin:** M. Mehdipour et al., "Rejuvenation of Three Germ Layers Tissues by Exchanging Old Blood Plasma with Saline-Albumin," *Aging* (Albany, NY) 12, no. 10 (May 2020): 8790–819.

263 convert adult cells back into embryonic stem cells: K. Takahashi and S. Yamanaka, "Induction of Pluripotent Stem Cells from Mouse Embryonic and Adult Fibroblast Cultures by Defined Factors," *Cell* 126, no. 4 (August 2006): 663–76.

264 used Yamanaka factors to reprogram the cells: Y. Lu et al., "Reprogramming to Recover Youthful Epigenetic Information and Restore Vision," *Nature* 588, no. 7836 (December 2020): 124–29.

264 reprogramming to delay or even reverse aging: A. Ocampo et al., "In Vivo Amelioration of Age-Associated Hallmarks by Partial Reprogramming," *Cell* 167, no. 7 (December 2016): 1719–33e12.

INDEX

Page numbers followed by *t* refer to tables.

telomeres
  measuring biological age with, 69–72
  and senescent cells, 52
  shortening of, in cell division, 50–51, 52,
    59, 70
  tracking length of, 113
TeloYears, 71
testosterone levels, 150
tests for biological age, consumer-based,
    34–35
Theranos, 77
therapeutic interventions for aging
  epigenetic reprogramming, 262–66
  and mTOR pathway, 252–55
  and pace of science progress, 251
  rapamycin and rapalogs, 253–55
  senolytics, 255–58
  young blood, 259–62
thymus, 197
thyroid issues, 218
time-restricted eating (TRE), 181–82,
    184–85
trans fats, 47
transposable elements, 49
triglycerides, 138–39, 157
tryptophan, 130, 165
Tufts University, 146
tumorigenesis, 13
23andMe, 106

ultramarathoners, 207
Unisom (doxylamine), 224
United Kingdom, 106
United States, gender paradox in, 96
University of Wisconsin, Madison (UW),
    138–41, 143
U.S. Food and Drug Administration (FDA),
    120–21

vaccines, 199
Van de Sluis, Bart, 256
Van Deursen, Jan, 256–57
vegan diet. See plant-based diet
vegetarian diet, 169, 170. See also
    plant-based diet
Venter, Craig, 118
Vilain, Eric, 79
Villeda, Saul, 200, 261
visceral fat, 159, 175

vitamin B12, 57
VO2 max, 193–94, 202, 204, 205

Wagers, Amy, 260
Walford, Lisa, 133
Walford, Roy, 133, 134–35, 136
walking, 202, 208
Ward, Peter, 117, 123–24
Washington Times, 15
Washington University, 146
weathering hypothesis, 243
weight, changes in
  and bariatric surgery, 157
  and caloric restriction, 153
  and Cushing's disease, 232
  and hormonal changes driving hunger,
    159–60
  and number of fat cells, 157, 159
Weismann, August, 50
Weissman, Irving, 260
Western diet, 141, 143, 145
white blood cells, 53–54, 75t
Wijshake, Tobias, 256
Wilks, James, 166
women
  and debilitating conditions, 96
  domestic/familial burdens carried by, 227–28
  and fat cells, 159
  and gender paradox, 95–99
  and menopause, 80, 83, 203
  and osteoporosis, 203
  in workforce, 226–27
work culture, 226–27
World Economic Forum, 240
World Health Organization (WHO), 203
World War II and Dutch Hunger Winter,
    241–42

Yale Cancer Center, 12
Yamanaka, Shinya, 262–63
Yamanaka factors, 263–65
yeast study, 102–5, 107, 110
young blood (therapeutic intervention), 259–62

Zhang, Kang, 79
Zhou, Daohong, 256
zip code as determinant of aging, 238
Zolman, Oliver, 246
Zone diet, 143